Clinician's Manual on
Myelodysplastic Syndromes

W0106212

REVLIMID® (lenalidomide) is indicated for the treatment of patients with transfusion-dependent anemia due to Low- or Intermediate-1-risk myelodysplastic syndromes associated with a deletion 5q cytogenetic abnormality, with or without additional cytogenetic abnormalities.

VIDAZA is indicated for treatment of patients with the following myelodysplastic syndrome subtypes: refractory anemia or refractory anemia with ringed sideroblasts (if accompanied by neutropenia or thrombocytopenia or requiring transfusions), refractory anemia with excess blasts, refractory anemia with excess blasts in transformation, and chronic myelomonocytic leukemia.

Clinician's Manual on
Myelodysplastic Syndromes

Alan List

Executive Vice President, Physician-in-Chief

H. Lee Moffitt Cancer Center & Research Institute

Tampa, FL

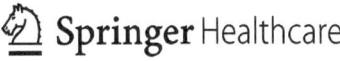 Springer Healthcare

Published by Springer Healthcare Ltd, 236 Gray's Inn Road, London, WC1X 8HB, UK

www.springerhealthcare.com

© 2008 Springer Healthcare, a part of Springer Science+Business Media

British Library Cataloguing-in-Publication Data.

A catalogue record for this book is available from the British Library.

ISBN 978-1-85873-427-9

Although every effort has been made to ensure that drug doses and other information are presented accurately in this publication, the ultimate responsibility rests with the prescribing physician. Neither the publisher nor the authors can be held responsible for errors or for any consequences arising from the use of the information contained herein. Any product mentioned in this publication should be used in accordance with the prescribing information prepared by the manufacturers. No claims or endorsements are made for any drug or compound at present under clinical investigation.

Project editor: Nadine Lemmens
Designer: Joe Harvey
Production: Marina Maher

Contents

Author biography

Dr Alan F. List is the Executive Vice President and Physician-in-Chief at the H. Lee Moffitt Cancer Center and Research Institute at the University of South Florida in Tampa, FL. After earning his bachelor and master of science degrees from Bucknell University, Dr List earned his medical degree at the University of Pennsylvania, College of Medicine. He completed fellowship training in medical oncology and in hematology at Vanderbilt University Medical Center. Dr List joined the University of Arizona Cancer Center in 1988, where, over his 17-year tenure, he served as Director of the Bone Marrow Transplant and Leukemia programs, and Deputy Director of Research before joining the Moffitt Cancer Center in 2003.

Dr List is internationally recognized for his work in the investigation of the biology and treatment of myelodysplastic syndromes (MDS) and acute myeloid leukemia (AML) and has been recognized as one of the "Best Doctors in America". He is a member of numerous professional societies, including the American Society of Hematology, American Society of Clinical Oncology, and the American Association for Cancer Research, and serves as an advisor for many pharmaceutical companies developing novel therapeutics for MDS and AML. Dr List serves as the Vice-Chair of the Leukemia Committee in the Southwest Oncology Group, and, in addition to roles as Associate Editor for several journals, he is a member of the Board of Directors of the MDS Foundation and the Aplastic Anemia & MDS International Foundation.

Author biography

Chapter 1

Introduction to myelodysplastic syndromes

Myelodysplastic syndromes (MDS) are a complex and heterogeneous group of malignancies of the multipotent hematopoietic stem cells [1–3]. Clinically and morphologically, MDS are characterized by dysplastic and ineffective hematopoiesis, resulting in peripheral blood cytopenias and an increased risk for transformation to AML. Despite an increased fraction of proliferating cells, MDS bone marrow progenitors display impaired differentiation potential, accelerated apoptosis (or programmed cell death), and, as a consequence, bone marrow failure (Figure 1.1). The net clinical result is ineffective hematopoiesis with intractable peripheral cytopenias: anemia, thrombocytopenia, and/or neutropenia.

Anemia, and its attendant symptoms of fatigue and weakness, is the most common cytopenia in MDS, affecting more than 80% of patients over time. At the time of diagnosis, 30% of patients have thrombocytopenia, and up to two-thirds of patients develop thrombocytopenia during the course of the disease [1,4,5]. Bleeding complications in those with thrombocytopenia range from mild petechiae and gingival bleeding to gastrointestinal bleeding and catastrophic intracranial hemorrhage.

White blood cell (WBC) abnormalities are present in approximately 50% of patients at the time of initial diagnosis [1]. Neutropenia and neutrophil dysfunction are common, increasing the risk for infection, which is the leading cause of death (see *Chapter 3*) [1–3]. MDS are also associated with a heightened risk of transformation to AML that varies depending upon disease features.

The vast majority of MDS cases (80–90%) occur *de novo* (primary MDS), and are of unknown etiology [1,6]. The risk increases with age, implicating hematopoietic senescence as a potential underlying cause. The disease can occur as a consequence of cumulative exposures to environmental genotoxins such as benzene, tobacco smoke, insecticides, and pesticides, as well as genetic susceptibilities and age-dependent loss of bone marrow

Figure 1.1 Characteristics of myelodysplastic syndromes

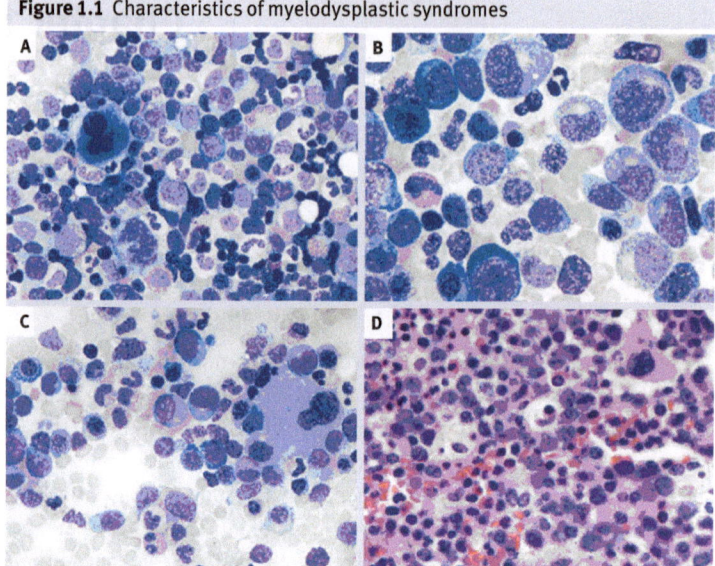

The bone marrow aspirate in patients with myelodysplasia of varied lineages of dysplasia often accompanied by a hypercellular biopsy (Panel A; Wright–Giemsa stain). In this specimen, hypolobated megakaryocytes and hyposegmented neutrophils are prominent. Myeloid maturation is impaired, and myeloblasts may be increased, as shown in Panel B in a patient with refractory anemia with excess blasts (Wright–Giemsa stain). Dyserythropoiesis accompanies the hypolobated megakaryocytes and hyposegmented neutrophils. There may be a left shift in erythroid maturation, with dysplastic features such as nuclear budding, megaloblastic changes, and as shown in Panel C, a decrease in the number of erythroid precursors (Wright–Giemsa stain). The cellularity of a core-biopsy specimen can approach 100%, with readily apparent dysplasia (Panel D; hematoxylin and eosin). Courtesy of Lynn Moscinski, M.D., H. Lee Moffitt Cancer Center and Research Institute, Tampa, FL.

function [1,6]. The remaining 10–20% of cases are considered secondary as they are directly associated with exposure to radiation and/or mutagenic chemotherapeutic agents, particularly alkylating agents. The risk of MDS following the completion of chemotherapy with alkylating agents may persist for up to 10 years [3].

Descriptions of the MDS have appeared in the medical literature for at least 70 years, with references ranging from refractory anemia, preleukemic anemia and smoldering acute leukemia, to hypoplastic acute myelogenous leukemia among others (Figure 1.2) [3,6]. The varied nosology reflects the varied pathogenetic features of the disease phenotype in MDS (see *Chapter 2*),

Figure 1.2 Historical terminology for myelodysplastic syndromes

Term	Year
Refractory anemia	1938
Preleukemic anemia	1949
Preleukemia	1953
Refractory anemia with ringed sideroblasts	1956
Refractory normoblastic anemia	1959
Smoldering acute leukemia	1963
Chronic erythremic myelosis	1969
Preleukemic syndrome	1973
Subacute myelomonocytic leukemia	1974
Chronic myelomonocytic leukemia	1974
Hypoplastic acute myelogenous leukemia	1975
Refractory anemia with excess myeloblasts	1976
Hematopoietic dysplasia	1978
Subacute myeloid leukemia	1979
Dysmyelopoietic syndrome	1980
Myelodysplastic syndromes	1982

Adapted with permission from List *et al.* [6].

the heterogeneous morphologic subtypes, and the range in disease severity (see *Chapter 5*). In 1982, an international group of researchers known as the French–American–British (FAB) Cooperative Group reported the first consensus morphologic classification system for MDS that recognized five major subgroups, which brought uniformity to the diagnosis and estimation of disease prognosis [7]. This classification system is still used in clinical practice today, although it is gradually being superseded by a more recent system recommended by the World Health Organization (WHO). This newer classification reflects advances in knowledge since publication of the FAB criteria, such as recognition of a cytogenetic subgroup for which specific treatments are now available (see *Chapter 6*) [3,8].

Like the disease itself, treatment options for MDS are variable, and are dependent upon the disease subtype and patients' individual risk profiles, age, and co-morbidities. Supportive treatments such as red blood cell (RBC) and platelet transfusions for symptomatic anemia and thrombocytopenia, iron chelation for patients with excessive iron owing to RBC transfusions, and erythropoietic growth factors are considered the standard of care for patients with MDS. However, new low- and high-intensity therapies are emerging, several of which have received approval from the US Food & Drug Administration (FDA) for the treatment of MDS [9,10]. The former treatments include biologic response modifiers (e.g., antithymocyte globulin [ATG], thalidomide, lenalidomide, and cyclosporine) and hypomethylating agents, and the latter induction chemotherapy and hematopoietic (marrow or peripheral blood) stem cell transplantation. Generally, low-intensity treatment with supportive care is recommended for lower risk patients, and high-intensity therapies, because of attendant risks of morbidity and mortality, are reserved for younger patients with higher risk disease [9,10].

Epidemiology

Given the historically varied terminology for MDS, it has been difficult to discern accurate estimates of the incidence and prevalence of the disease. Historical estimates of the annual incidence of *de novo* MDS range from 2 to 5 cases per 100,000 population, and indicate that incidence increases with age [1,10]. There are an estimated 22–45 cases per 100,000 among those over 70 years of age, and more than 80% of MDS patients are more than 60 years old [1,3,10]. Onset before age 50 is uncommon and more often associated with mutagen exposure. In the US, it is estimated that between 30,000 and 50,000 persons are living with the disease [3].

The most recent and definitive epidemiologic evidence to date are drawn from the Surveillance, Epidemiology, and End Results (SEER) program, a national cancer registry sponsored by the National Cancer Institute, which began collecting data on MDS in 2001 [11]. The registry is considered the definitive source on the incidence of many types of cancer in the US. Data on the incidence of MDS are available for the years 2001 to 2003, and were collected in 17 regions in the US, capturing a population of more than 76 million people.

During this time period, an annual total of 7131 cases of MDS were made. Median age at diagnosis was 76 years, 86% of cases were more than 60 years old, and the incidence increased with age for both genders (Figure 1.3) [11]. MDS was more common in men than women. The age-adjusted incidence in men was 4.5 per 100,000 per year (95% confidence interval [CI] 4.3–4.6 per 100,000 per year) versus 2.7 per 100,000 per year in women (95% CI, 2.6–2.8 per 100,000). When the data were analyzed by race, whites had the highest incidence, and native American-Indians, Alaska Natives, and Asian-Pacific Islanders the lowest. When the 2003 incidence rate, adjusted for age, gender, and race, was applied to the entire US population, the overall rate was estimated at 10,351 cases per year [11].

Figure 1.3 Age-specific incidence rates of myelodysplastic syndromes in the US (2001–2003)

Age (years)	Men and women		Men		Women	
	Count	Rate*	Count	Rate*	Count	Rate*
0	8	0.2	3	0.2	5	0.3
1–4	26	0.2	13	0.2	13	0.2
5–9	10	0.1	2	0	8	0.1
10–14	12	0.1	5	0.1	7	0.1
15–19	17	0.1	8	0.1	9	0.1
20–24	12	0.1	9	0.1	3	0
25–29	18	0.1	11	0.1	7	0.1
30–34	30	0.2	22	0.3	8	0.1
35–39	58	0.3	33	0.4	25	0.3
40–44	100	0.6	56	0.6	44	0.5
45–49	148	0.9	72	0.9	76	0.9
50–54	216	1.5	112	1.6	104	1.4
55–59	314	2.8	161	2.9	153	2.6
60–64	460	5.4	257	6.3	203	4.6
65–69	686	10	386	12.2	300	8.1
70–74	1032	16.6	599	21.8	433	12.6
75–79	1374	25.7	785	35.7	589	18.7
80–84	1406	36.2	729	48.9	677	28.3
≥85	1204	36.4	565	54.7	639	28
Total	7131	–	3828	–	3303	–

*Rates are per 100,000 per year. Data from the Surveillance, Epidemiology, and End Results (SEER) program. Reproduced with permission from Ma *et al.* [11].

Risk factors

Few risk factors for *de novo* MDS have been identified. These include age, gender, heredity, genetics, and exposure to environmental toxins.

Age: Although MDS can and do occur in children, childhood onset is rare. When it occurs in the pediatric setting, median age of onset is 6 years [6]. Pediatric MDS tends to follow a similar clinical course to adult disease, with peripheral cytopenias and their accompanying conditions. MDS in children is often associated with monosomy of chromosome 7 [1]. Nevertheless, MDS is predominantly a disease of the elderly, with the incidence increasing dramatically after age 60. *De novo* disease is uncommon in younger individuals.

Gender: Men have a higher risk for MDS than women [1,11].

Heredity: A familial predisposition to MDS has been reported for isolated younger cases, but appears to be rare [3,12,13].

Genetics: The pathogenesis of MDS may begin with acquisition of a genetic change that disrupts stem cell function and maturation potential, resulting in the proliferation of an abnormal clone. Genetic conditions such as Fanconi's anemia, Shwachman–Diamond Syndrome, Down's syndrome, neurofibromatosis, and mitochondrial cytopathies have also been associated with a predisposition to MDS [1].

Environmental toxins: Exposure to benzene, cigarette smoke, pesticides, and insecticides is associated with MDS [1,6,14].

Treatment-related MDS: Secondary MDS has been observed following treatment with antineoplastic agents (particularly alkylating agents) and autologous bone marrow transplantation [1].

Prognosis

The disease course and prognosis of MDS are variable and range from indolent to aggressive. Estimates of survival range from 5 months to years depending on the type of MDS and individual patient characteristics. According to the SEER registry, the 3-year survival rate is 42%, and men are 25% more likely to die than women [11]. Important prognostic variables include age, gender, the percentage of bone marrow blasts, karyotype [good: diploid, -y, isolated del(5q), del(20q); poor: chromosome 7 abnormalities or ≥3 complex abnormalities], the number of cytopenias, and RBC transfusion dependence (Figure 1.4) [11,15].

Because MDS is almost exclusively a disease of the elderly, most patients will suffer from multiple co-morbidities. Factors such as previous cancers, heart disease, diabetes mellitus, and other chronic conditions will influence treatment decisions and impact survival. Some patients may be unable to endure high-intensity treatments, and others will ultimately succumb to other medical conditions, not MDS itself [6,16].

Figure 1.4 Prognostic factors in myelodysplastic syndrome

Leukemia burden
French–American–British (FAB) type
Abnormal localization of immature precursors
In vitro culture pattern
Fraction CD34+ cells

Lineage penetrance and severity of maturation impairment
Number of cytopenias
Number of dysplastic lineages
Cytopenia severity

Genetic abnormalities
Cytogenetic pattern
DNA ploidy
Protooncogene mutations
Epigenetic gene silencing

Clinical and pathologic features
De novo versus therapy-related myelodysplastic syndrome
RBC transfusion dependence
Bone marrow fibrosis
Abnormal localization of immature precursors

RBC, red blood cell. Adapted with permission from List *et al.* [6].

The risk of transformation to AML varies, depending on the MDS subtype and karyotype, and ranges from approximately 10% to more than 50% [1,10]. Patients with AML that arise from MDS (AML-MDS), as compared to those with *de novo* AML, are often more resistant to standard AML treatment regimens, and survival is generally short following disease transformation [10,17].

Chapter 2

Etiology and pathophysiology

The precise etiology of *de novo* MDS is unknown. The disease has been associated with exposure to environmental toxins, such as benzene, and therapeutic radiation, with some evidence, albeit limited, supporting genetic predisposition in younger individuals. Secondary disease is specifically associated with cytoxic chemotherapy. The principal contributing factor may also be associated with intrinsic aging processes [6].

There are two fundamental features of the pathobiology of MDS: excessive apoptosis of stem cell progeny and impaired blood cell maturation [2,6,18]. The disease process is believed to arise from a genetic injury in hematopoietic stem cells. Such genetic lesions may be introduced either by exposure to some type of environmental or chemical toxin, a hematopoietic senescence, or other etiology. The mutated stem cells then proliferate, and, eventually, the abnormal clones dominate the bone marrow and suppress healthy stem cells.

The clonal proliferation of myelodysplastic hematopoietic stem cells culminates in ineffective hematopoiesis characterized by excessive apoptosis of maturing cells. The MDS are not diseases of suppressed or insufficient hematopoiesis; they are conditions of ineffective hematopoiesis. A non-productive cycling of blood cell progenitors and impaired cell maturation ensues [6,18,19]. Over time, peripheral cytopenias that typify MDS arise.

This apparent paradox of bone marrow hypercellularity and peripheral blood cytopenias is accompanied by excess generation of a variety of cytokines including angiogenic molecules, such as vascular endothelial growth factor, and pro-inflammatory cytokines that promote apoptosis, such as tumor necrosis factor (TNF)-α, interleukin (IL)-1β, IL-6, transforming growth factor-β, and soluble Fas ligand [3,20]. As the disease progresses, the maturation potential of the clone may worsen with progression to more aggressive disease, and transformation to acute myeloid leukemia (AML).

Multiple cytogenetic abnormalities – similar to those that occur in AML of the elderly – may contribute to the development of MDS, and are found in 50–60% of patients with *de novo* MDS and 75–85% of patients with secondary disease [1–3,10,21]. Certain chromosomal abnormalities are particularly common [21]. The complete or partial loss of chromosome 5, for example, is found in 15% of patients with MDS, and the complete or partial loss of chromosome 7 is found in 5% of patients [15]. Trisomy 8 is found in 5% of patients, del20q in 2%, del17p in less than 1%, and a loss of X or Y occurs in about 2% of patients [15]. Also implicated are mutations in the *ras* oncogenes, the p53 and perhaps other tumor-suppressor genes, accompanied by deregulation of the anti-apoptotic *BCL2* gene, $p15^{INK4b}$, a cell-cycle inhibitor, and the transcript factor genes *EVI1* and *MLL* through promoter hypermethylation [2,21–23].

Chapter 3

Signs and symptoms of myelodysplastic syndromes

The symptoms of MDS – both *de novo* and secondary – are nonspecific and largely dependent on the type and severity of the underlying cytopenia. In the early stages of disease, patients are often asymptomatic and a diagnosis of MDS is discovered incidentally during a routine blood analysis. In the later stages of disease, patients may present with symptoms of anemia, neutropenia or thrombocytopenia, or some combination. In fact, at least one-half of patients have pancytopenia at the time of diagnosis [6]. The severity of symptoms and disease manifestations, which range from mild to life-threatening, adversely affect the patient's quality of life (QoL) [4,24,25].

Anemia
Anemia is the most frequently observed cytopenia in patients with MDS, affecting more than 80% of patients [25]. The signs and symptoms of MDS-associated anemia mimic those of other types of anemias. Typical symptoms result from tissue hypoxia associated with a decline in hemoglobin <10 g/dL and may include:
- fatigue, weakness, irritability;
- dyspnea, particularly on exertion;
- chest pain;
- palpitations;
- headache, dizziness (particularly postural) and vertigo;
- tinnitus;
- syncope;
- difficulty sleeping or concentrating;
- anorexia; and
- decreased libido or impotence.

There may be physical findings in multiple parts of the body:
- **Skin:** Pale or purpura or petechiae may be present.
- **Eyes:** Pale conjunctiva, retinal hemorrhages.
- **Cardiovascular:** Tachycardia, orthostatic hypotension.
- **Pulmonary:** Tachypnea, rales.
- **Abdomen:** Hepatomegaly and/or splenomegaly.
- **Neurologic:** Peripheral neuropathy, difficulty with concentration.

Neutropenia

Neutropenia is characterized by an absolute neutrophil count of less than 1500 cells/mm^3, and often occurs in the presence of anemia. Approximately 50% of patients are neutropenic at the time of diagnosis, and approximately 20% of patients report an increased incidence of infection [1,25]. Neutropenia itself may be asymptomatic, but infections vary. Bacterial skin infections are the most common, although other sites are possible, as are fungal infections [26,27]. Bacterial infections typically respond poorly to antimicrobial therapy [6]. Infections are the leading cause of death among patients with MDS [6,26].

Thrombocytopenia

Thrombocytopenia, defined as a platelet count of less than 100×10^9/L, rarely occurs in the absence of anemia. Few MDS patients – less than 10% – initially present with serious bleeding [4]. However, as many as two-thirds of patients with MDS eventually suffer from thrombocytopenia [4] and at least 80% suffer from some degree of platelet dysfunction resulting in decreased aggregation [5]. The incidence of thrombocytopenia and severe thrombocytopenia (platelet count less than 20×10^9/L) varies across FAB subtypes, and the incidence appears to increase with increasing disease risk (Figure 3.1) [4].

The bleeding events that result from MDS-related thrombocytopenia vary in location, severity, and consequence [28]. Minor events include petechiae, gingival bleeding, and trauma-related hematoma, with more serious events ranging from gastrointestinal hemorrhage to intracranial, retinal, and pulmonary hemorrhage. No exact statistics are available on the actual incidence of these events in MDS patients; however, it has been estimated that 3–5% of MDS patients experience intracranial hemorrhage, 6–7% gastrointestinal hemorrhage, and 18% some type of moderate-to-severe hemorrhagic event [4]. Bleeding events are reported as direct contributors to death in 10–24% of patients with MDS [28].

Figure 3.1 Incidence of thrombocytopenia and severe thrombocytopenia according to FAB subtype and IPSS classification in 2410 patients

	Total number	Thrombocytopenia (%)*	Severe thrombocytopenia (%)†
FAB classification			
Refractory anemia (RA)	577	58	15
Refractory anemia with ringed sideroblasts (RARS)	175	43	13
Refractory anemia with excess blasts (RAEB)	804	71	17
Refractory anemia with excess blasts in transformation (RAEB-t)	680	77	22
Chronic myelomonocytic leukemia (CMML)	174	55	10
IPSS group			
Primary untreated			
Low risk	257	20	2
Intermediate-1 risk	603	64	15
Intermediate-2 risk	514	72	16
High risk	382	82	25
Secondary MDS‡	507	75	21
Prior chemotherapy‡	76	73	22

*Platelet count <100 x 10⁹/L; †Platelet count <20 x 10⁹/L; ‡Patients in these groups could not be categorized using the International Prognosis Scoring System (IPSS) because the system excludes secondary MDS and prior chemotherapy. FAB, French–American–British. Adapted from Kantarjian *et al.* [4].

Cutaneous manifestations of MDS

Cutaneous manifestations of MDS are typically rare, with two exceptions: Sweet's syndrome and granulocytic sarcoma. In Sweet's syndrome (also known as acute febrile neutrophilic dermatosis), patients develop recurring fever accompanied by painful or tender erythematosus papules and plaques in the upper dermis (Figure 3.2) [29]. On histopathology, it is characterized by a dense infiltrate of neutrophils. When occurring *de novo*, it indicates a diagnosis of MDS, and, in established patients, it may herald disease acceleration [30,31]. Corticosteroids are usually the treatment of choice [29,30,32].

Granulocytic sarcoma is an infiltration of the dermis and subcutaneous tissue of immature myeloblasts (Figure 3.3) [33]. It, too, is often an indication of acceleration of disease [6,31].

Figure 3.2 Clinical and histologic aspects in "initial" lymphocytic and "late" neutrophilic Sweet syndrome

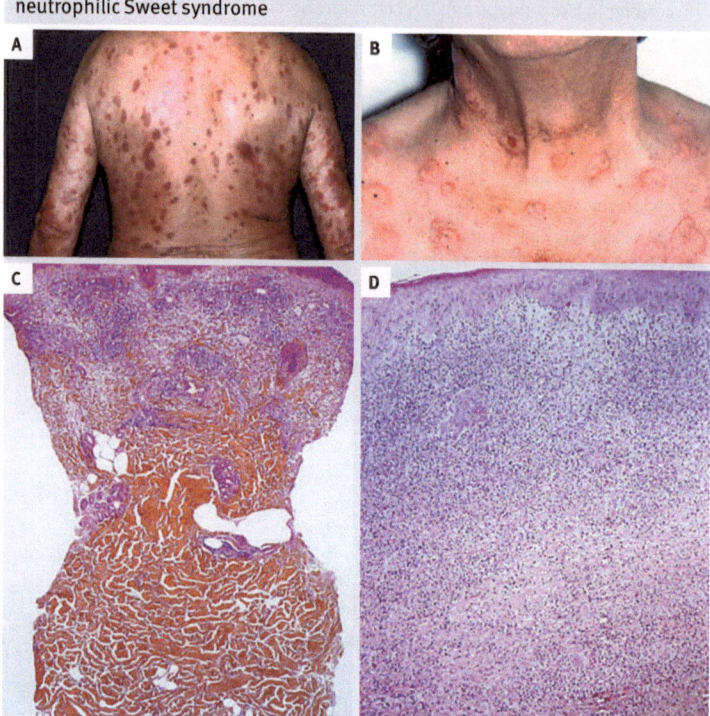

(A) Disseminated erythematous plaques over the trunk and arms.
(B) Erythematous plaques with annular configuration. (C) Dense lymphocytic infiltrates located in the superficial and middermis (hematoxylin-eosin, original magnification x10). (D) Massive dermal neutrophilic infiltrates without vasculitis (hematoxylin-eosin, original magnification x20). Reproduced with permission from Vignon-Pennamen *et al.* [30].

Ocular manifestations of MDS

Ocular manifestations of MDS may occur in as many as 46% of patients, but often go unrecognized [35]. These complications may include corneal ulcer, iridocyclitis, vitreous hemorrhage, retinal hemorrhage, cotton wool spots, and optic neuritis, and multiple ocular complications may be present in a single patient. Reduced platelet counts are associated with a risk for retinal hemorrhage. The incidence of ocular complications appears to be higher in the subgroup of patients with refractory anemia with excess blasts than in the subgroup with refractory anemia alone [35].

Figure 3.3 Granulocytic sarcoma

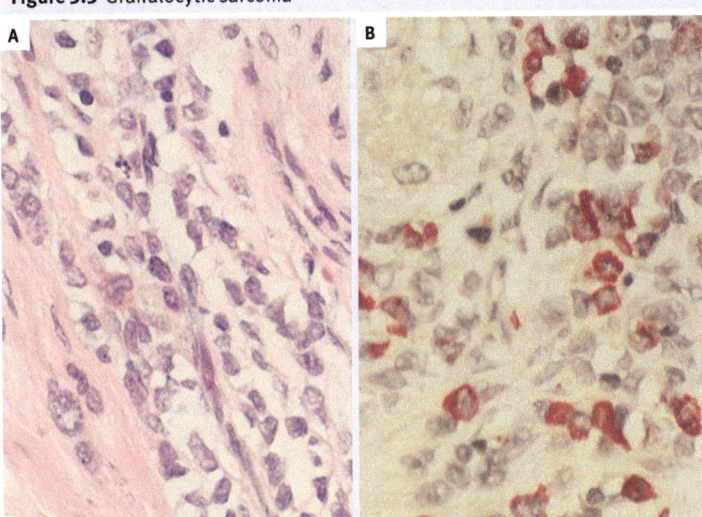

Granulocytic sarcoma is a rare condition of the cervix. (A) Some large cells with red granular cytoplasm can be seen, which appear to be eosinophilic myelocytes. (B) A Leder (chloroacetate esterase) stain highlights (red) the granules typical of myeloid differentiation. Reproduced with permission from Stenchever & Goff [34].

Splenomegaly and hepatomegaly in MDS

Splenic or hepatic enlargements are uncommon in MDS, with the specific exception of the chronic myelomonocytic leukemia (CMML) subtype. The current WHO classification system considers CMML a hybrid disorder with both myelodysplastic and myeloproliferative features that is distinct from more conventional MDS (see *Chapter 5*) [8].

Impact on quality of life

The symptoms of MDS have a definite and adverse effect on patients' QoL [24,25]. A recent internet survey of 359 patients with MDS assessed QoL using several validated QoL instruments, and compared results in MDS patients with those of the general population [25]. Overall, MDS patients consistently scored worse on these instruments than their healthy counterparts. The most common and disruptive symptoms as reported by patients were fatigue (89%), bruising/bleeding (55%), night sweats (43%), bone pain (39%), fevers (28%), skin rashes (25%), undesired weight loss (25%), and recurrent infections (20%) [25].

Of the survey respondents, 30% also reported that they were unable to work outside the home because of MDS-related symptoms, and another 5% claimed some other type of disability [25]. The symptoms and manifestations of MDS are potentially serious and debilitating.

Chapter 4

Clinical assessment and diagnosis

The diagnosis of *de novo* and secondary MDS is based on morphologic findings in the peripheral blood and bone marrow in patients with cytopenias. As a variety of diseases and conditions may cause anemia and other cytopenias, tests are required to exclude these and confirm the presence of MDS (Figure 4.1), and to delineate patients' prognoses. Each of these factors is an important consideration when developing a treatment strategy. Recommended investigations include [10]:

- history (including documentation of toxic exposure and transfusion history);
- complete blood cell count, including platelets, WBC differential, and reticulocytes;
- examination of peripheral blood smear;
- bone marrow aspiration with iron stain and biopsy;
- bone marrow cytogenetics;
- serum erythropoietin (EPO) level (in the presence of anemia);
- RBC folate and serum B_{12}; and
- serum ferritin ± iron, total iron binding capacity.

Figure 4.1 Differentials in myelodysplastic syndromes

Agranulocytosis

Anemia of chronic disease

Aplastic anemia

Bone marrow failure

Chronic myelogenous leukemia

Hairy cell leukemia

Megaloblastic anemia

Myelophthisic anemia

Myeloproliferative disease

Red cell aplasia

Results of these evaluations are correlated with the FAB [7] and WHO [8] classification criteria to establish a specific MDS diagnosis and prognosis [10]. Specifically, these morphologic classification systems base diagnosis on the percentage of blasts in the peripheral blood and bone marrow, and the presence or absence of ringed sideroblasts or monocytosis (see *Chapter 5*).

History

Patient history is important for establishing the timing, severity, and history of symptomatic cytopenias, and establishing a patient's baseline health, QoL, and functional status. Each of these factors are considered when determining the risk–benefit ratio of low- and high-intensity therapy for individual patients [10]. Patients should be questioned about past infections and bleeding events, as well as about anemia symptoms and past transfusions, and their current QoL. The majority of MDS patients are elderly, and are therefore likely to be suffering from another chronic ailment, and to be taking one or more medications, either of which may be an underlying cause of anemia. A thorough medical history will also help to exclude other possible causes of anemia and other cytopenias.

Complete blood cell counts

MDS evolves relatively slowly. Therefore, establishing a baseline blood cell count and monitoring temporal changes is necessary for establishing disease severity and progression risk [10].

Peripheral blood smears

Peripheral blood smears are necessary to establish the existence of cytopenias, and to determine which lineages are dysplastic and the degree of dysplasia. Smears may reveal a variety of abnormalities.

- **RBC changes:** Anemia, the most frequently identified abnormality in MDS, is defined as a hemoglobin concentration less than 10 g/dL. It is most often macrocytic or normocytic, with oval-shaped RBC (macro-ovalocytes). Mean corpuscular volume is typically less than 120 μm^3. Other changes may include irregularly or elliptically shaped red cells, red cells of different sizes, or stomatocytes. Low reticulocyte counts are common, and stippled or nucleated red cells are occasionally observed.
- **WBC changes:** WBC counts range from normal to low in patients with MDS and approximately 50% have neutropenia on diagnosis. Monocytes may be increased (levels greater than 1 x 10^9/L defines CMML). Morphologic changes in the granulocytes may include bilobed or unsegmented nuclei

(pseudo-Pelger–Huët abnormality), and decreased granulation. Bactericidal activity may be impaired and renders patients at increased risk of infection. Decreased numbers of natural killer T cells and helper T lymphocytes are a common finding.

- **Platelet changes:** At the time of diagnosis, approximately 30% of MDS patients have thrombocytopenia with dysplastic features such as hypogranulation and megakaryocyte fragments. Aggregation is decreased.

Bone marrow aspiration and biopsy

Bone marrow aspiration and biopsy is recommended for every patient with suspected MDS [1,10]. These tests are needed to evaluate the extent of abnormalities in hematopoietic cell maturation, the percentage of marrow blasts, marrow cellularity, and the presence of iron and ringed sideroblasts, fibrosis, and cytogenetic abnormalities. Common morphologic abnormalities are shown in Figure 4.2. In most patients (85–90%) the marrow is normo- or hypercellular with more than one lineage of dysplasia [1,10]. For a diagnosis of MDS, the WHO requires detection of cytologic dysplasia in 10% or more of cells from any affected lineage [8].

Other changes may include vitamin B_{12} or folate deficiencies, and bi- or multinuclear erythroid precursors. WBC dysplasias (dysmyelopoiesis) may include impaired myeloid maturation with elevated myeloblast, myelocyte, and metamyelocyte counts, and myeloid hyperplasia. Abnormalities in the platelet lineage may include giant platelets or micromegakaryocytes or megakaryocytes with dispersed nuclei.

Marrow cytogenetic analysis

As cytogenetic abnormalities are found at baseline in 50–60% of patients with *de novo* MDS and 75–85% of those with secondary disease, and cytogenetic abnormalities are closely correlated with prognosis, guidelines recommend marrow cytogenetic analysis for all patients [10]. Common cytogenic abnormalities include the 5q deletion, monosomy 7 (–7) or 7q deletion, and trisomy 8 (+8) [21]. Figure 4.3 shows common abnormalities according to FAB classification and median survival. Specific therapy is available for MDS patients with the chromosome 5q deletion (see *Chapter 6*).

Additional tests and findings

Additional tests that may help facilitate the diagnosis and identify MDS treatment strategies include serum EPO, vitamin B_{12}, and RBC folate measurements. Serum ferritin levels may be increased, as well as concentrations of lactic dehydrogenase and uric acid. For patients with severe thrombocytopenia

Figure 4.2 Morphologic manifestations of myelodysplasia

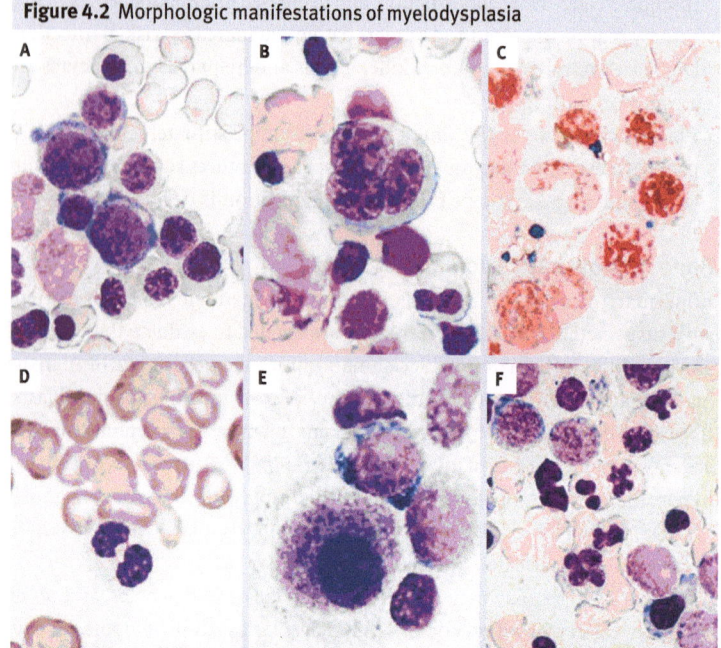

(A) Megaloblastic erythropoiesis with cytoplasmic blebbing in a bone marrow specimen (Wright–Giemsa stain, x100). (B) A multinucleated erythroid precursor in a bone marrow specimen (Wright–Giemsa stain, x100). (C) A ringed sideroblast in a bone marrow specimen (Prussian blue stain, x100). (D) A pseudo-Pelger–Huët neutrophil in a specimen of peripheral blood (Wright–Giemsa stain, x100). (E) A bone marrow micromegakaryocyte (Wright–Giemsa stain, x100). (F) Misshapen nuclei in bone marrow erythroid precursors (Wright–Giemsa stain, x100). Reproduced with permission from Heaney & Golde [3].

Figure 4.3 Karyotypic abnormalities in patient with myelodysplastic syndromes

FAB subgroup	Chromosomal abnormalities (%)	Frequently associated karyotypes	Median survival (months)
Refractory anemia	30	5q−, −7, +8, 20q−	32
Refractory anemia with ringed sideroblasts	20	+8, 5q−, 20q−	42
Refractory anemia with excess blasts	45	−7, 7q−, −5, 5q−, +8	12
Refractory anemia with excess blasts in transformation	60	−7, 7q−, −5, 5q−, +8	5
Chronic myelomonocytic leukemia	30	−7, +8, t(5;12), 7q−, 12q−	20

Reproduced with permission from Cortes *et al.* [1].

requiring platelet transfusion, human leukocyte antigen (HLA) typing may be helpful, and screening for cytomegalovirus in candidates for hematopoietic stem cell transplantation (HSCT) is also recommended [10].

Chapter 5

Classification of myelodysplastic syndromes

In 1982, the first morphologic classification system of MDS was reported [7]. The system, known as the French–American–British (FAB) classification, proved to be very useful in clinical practice, and continues to be widely used today by clinicians to determine the risk of transformation to AML and predict survival.

More recently, the WHO refined and updated the FAB classification in an effort to improve the clinical relevance of the subtypes and improve prognostic utility [8]. The WHO standard is gradually being adopted in clinical practice, and both systems are currently used in tandem with the International Prognostic Scoring System (IPSS) to determine the patient's disease risk, to assess the probability of transformation to AML, and to guide treatment decisions. Both morphologic systems are applicable to patients with *de novo* and secondary MDS, whereas IPSS is relevant only to *de novo* MDS.

The French–American–British classification

The FAB classification system identified five MDS subgroups, and distinguished these groups from AML. The distinctions are based on the percentage of blast cells in the peripheral blood and bone marrow, morphologic features of blast cells derived from bone marrow aspirates, and the presence or absence of ringed sideroblasts or monocytosis [7]. The FAB subgroups include (Figure 5.1):

- refractory anemia (RA);
- refractory anemia with ringed sideroblasts (RARS);
- refractory anemia with excess blasts (RAEB);
- refractory anemia with excess blasts in transformation (RAEB-t); and
- chronic myelomonocytic leukemia (CMML).

Figure 5.1 The FAB classification of MDS

FAB subtype	Peripheral blasts (%)	Bone marrow blasts (%)
Refractory anemia (RA)	<1	<5
Refractory anemia with ringed sideroblasts (RARS)	<1	<5
Refractory anemia with excess blasts (RAEB)	<5	5–20
Refractory anemia with excess blasts in transformation (RAEB-t)	≥5	21–30
Chronic myelomonocytic leukemia (CMML) (>1000 monocytes µg/L blood)	<5	5–20

FAB, French–American–British. Adapted from Bennett *et al.* [7].

Refractory anemia

Refractory anemia is defined as absence of blasts in the peripheral blood and less than 5% blasts in the bone marrow in patients with a normo- or hyper-cellular bone marrow, and evidence of dysplasia and cytopenia (usually anemia) in at least one lineage in the peripheral blood (Figure 5.2) [7]. It accounts for 10–40% of MDS diagnoses. RA typically has a more indolent clinical course with a median survival of 30–65 months, and a low

Figure 5.2 Refractory anemia

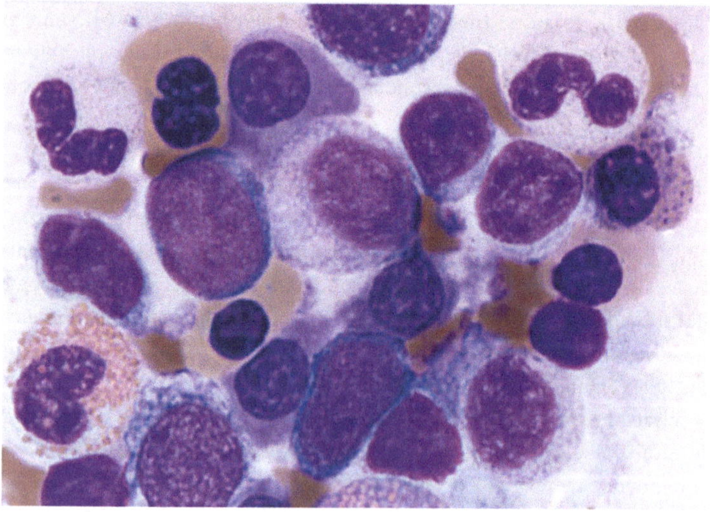

Courtesy of Lynn Moscinski, M.D., H. Lee Moffitt Cancer Center and Research Institute, Tampa, FL.

risk of progression to AML. The most recent data from the Surveillance, Epidemiology, and End Results (SEER) program indicate a median survival of 28 months [11].

Refractory anemia with ringed sideroblasts

FAB criteria for RARS include the same blast and cellularity requirements as for RA, but with the additional feature of the presence of ringed sideroblasts comprising more than 15% of all nucleated bone marrow erythroid cells (Figure 5.3) [7]. Like RA patients, RARS patients have a prolonged clinical course with median survival estimates ranging from 34 to 83 months, and a relatively low risk of transformation of AML. Between 10% and 25% of MDS diagnoses fall into this subgroup [11].

Refractory anemia with excess blasts

This MDS subgroup is defined as having less than 5% blasts in the peripheral blood and between 5% and 20% blasts in the bone marrow (Figure 5.4) [7]. Dysplasia is often evident in all three blood cell lineages with accompanying

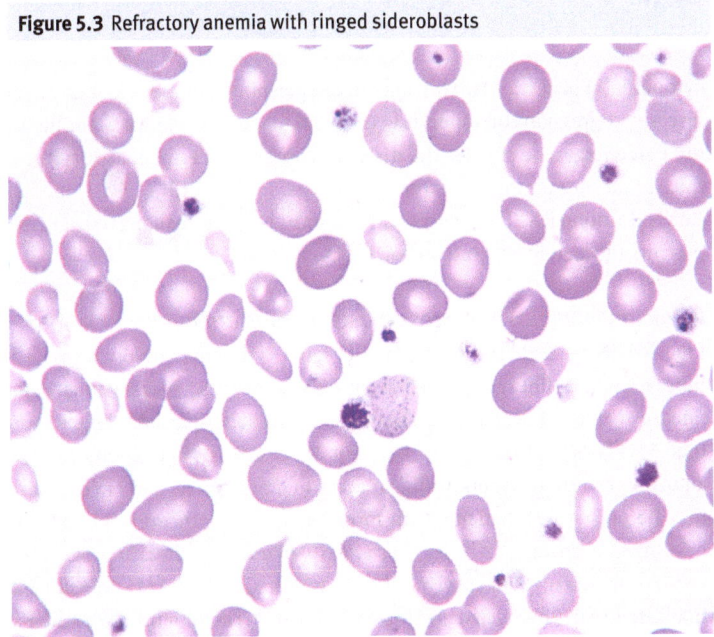

Figure 5.3 Refractory anemia with ringed sideroblasts

Courtesy of Lynn Moscinski, M.D., H. Lee Moffitt Cancer Center and Research Institute, Tampa, FL.

Figure 5.4 Refractory anemia with excess blasts

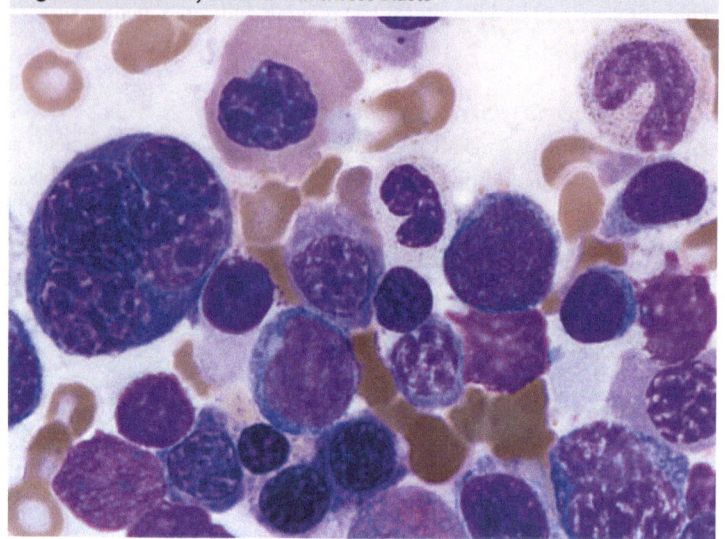

Courtesy of Lynn Moscinski, M.D., H. Lee Moffitt Cancer Center and Research Institute, Tampa, FL.

cytopenia(s) in at least two lineages in the peripheral blood. The rapidity of disease progression corresponds to the percentage of myeloblasts: the higher the percentage, the shorter the disease's course with a median survival in this subgroup ranging from 8 to 18 months. In the SEER registry, median survival among RAEB patients was 11 months [11]. More than 50% of RAEB patients ultimately progress to AML.

Refractory anemia with excess blasts in transformation

Like RAEB patients, RAEB-t patients have cytopenias involving two or more blood cell lineages, as well as dysplastic changes generally in all three lineages (Figure 5.5). However, patients in this subgroup have either more than 5% blasts in the peripheral blood or 21–29% blasts in the bone marrow, and Auer rods (a red staining, linear array of granular material) in the blasts may be present [7]. Patients with more than 30% blasts are considered to have AML according to FAB criteria. Also, like RAEB, disease progression is rapid, with a median survival of 4–11 months, and an AML transformation rate of 50–90%. Between 10% and 30% of MDS patients are estimated to have this MDS subtype.

Figure 5.5 Refractory anemia with excess blasts in transformation

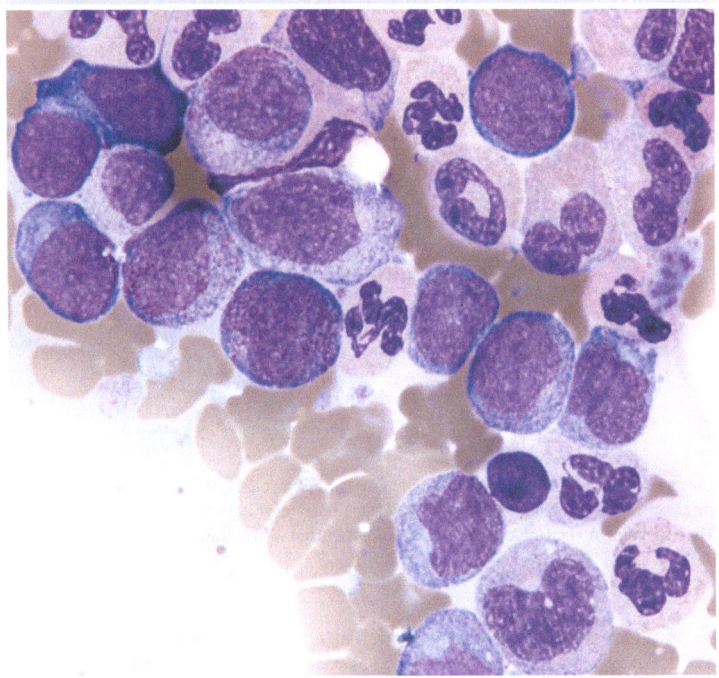

Courtesy of Lynn Moscinski, M.D., H. Lee Moffitt Cancer Center and Research Institute, Tampa, FL.

Chronic myelomonocytic leukemia

CMML is characterized by a peripheral blood monocyte count greater than $1x10^9$ cells/L (monocytosis), less than 5% blasts in the peripheral blood, and 20% or less blasts in the bone marrow (Figure 5.6) [7]. More than 40% of CMML patients progress to AML, and median survival is estimated at 15–32 months [7]. This subgroup accounts for approximately 10–20% of MDS diagnoses. Many clinicians consider CMML as an independent condition separate from the other MDS because it often has proliferative features such as leukocytosis that may more closely resemble a myeloproliferative condition than conventional myelodysplasia [2,3,37].

The WHO classification system

The WHO classification system of MDS is summarized in Figure 5.7 [8]. It includes many of the categories and concepts in the FAB system, but with

Figure 5.6 Mature monocytosis in chronic myelomonocytic leukemia

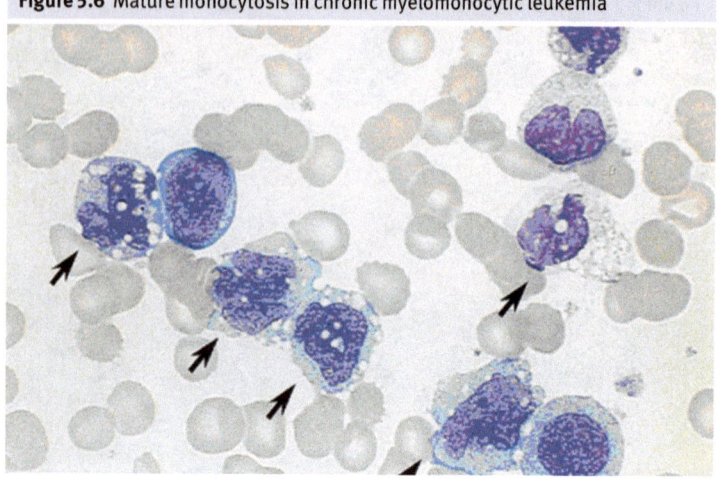

This peripheral blood smear from a patient with chronic myelomonocytic leukemia shows the mature monocytosis (arrows) that characterizes this disorder. (Wright-Giemsa stain, original magnification 100×). Reproduced with permission from Sobecks & Theil [36].

several important refinements, which attempt to address some ambiguities in the FAB criteria.

AML threshold

The threshold for diagnosis of AML was lowered from more than 30% blasts in the peripheral blood or bone marrow to 20%. This change eliminated the RAEB-t category of the FAB classification. The rationale behind this change was based on findings indicating that patients with RAEB-t and MDS-related AML share several important clinical and biological features.

Studies comparing RAEB-t and MDS-related AML found that these diseases have nearly identical proliferation and apoptosis profiles, and that these profiles differ markedly from RA, RARS, and RAEB [8]. RAEB-t and AML also share abnormalities in chromosome 7, heightened levels of multidrug-resistant glycoproteins, and suboptimal responses to chemotherapy. In fact, patients with biologically similar RAEB-t and AML treated with the same regimens have similar responses and survival times. Finally, the decision to lower the AML threshold was also based on findings that RAEB-t is an aggressive disease, with a greater than 60% risk of transformation to AML within 1 year, and a median survival time of less than 12 months [8,15].

Figure 5.7 The WHO classification and criteria for myelodysplastic syndromes

Disease	Blood findings	Bone marrow findings
Refractory anemia (RA)	Anemia No or rare blasts	Erythroid dysplasia only <5% blasts <15% ringed sideroblasts
Refractory anemia with ringed sideroblasts (RARS)	Anemia No blasts	Erythroid dysplasia only <5% blasts ≥15% ringed sideroblasts
Refractory cytopenia with multilineage dysplasia (RCMD)	Cytopenias (bicytopenia or pancytopenia) No or rare blasts No Auer rods <1 x 10⁹/L monocytes	Dysplasia in ≥10% of cells in 2 or more myeloid cell lines <5% blasts in marrow <15% ringed sideroblasts No Auer rods
Refractory cytopenia with multilineage dysplasia and ringed sideroblasts (RCMD-RS)	Cytopenias (bicytopenia or pancytopenia) No or rare blasts No Auer rods <1 x 10⁹/L monocytes	Dysplasia in ≥10% of cells in 2 or more myeloid cell lines <5% blasts ≥15% ringed sideroblasts No Auer rods
Refractory anemia with excess blasts-1 (RAEB-1)	Cytopenias <5% blasts No Auer rods <1 x 10⁹/L monocytes	Unilineage or multilineage dysplasia 5–9% blasts No Auer rods
Refractory anemia with excess blasts-2 (RAEB-2)	Cytopenias <5% blasts Auer rods ± <1 x 10⁹/L monocytes	Unilineage or multilineage dysplasia 10–19% blasts Auer rods ±
MDS associated with isolated del(5q)	Anemia <5% blasts Platelets normal or increased	Normal to megakaryocytes with hypolobated nuclei <5% blasts No Auer rods Isolated del(5q)
MDS, unclassified (MDS-U)	Cytopenias No or rare blasts No Auer rods	Unilineage dysplasia in granulocytes or megakaryocytes <5% blasts No Auer rods

Reproduced with permission from Vardiman et al. [8].

Refining refractory anemia

The original FAB definitions of RA and RARS included patients with erythroid-only dysplasia as well as patients with more severe multilineage dysplasia [7]. Subsequent studies have shown that there are substantial differences in disease characteristics and prognosis between single lineage and multilineage dysplasias [38,39].

Patients with erythroid-only dysplasia tend to develop symptoms limited to anemia, whereas those with multilineage dysplasia may also develop symptoms of granulocyte and platelet abnormalities (e.g., infection and bleeding). In addition, when compared to patients with multilineage disease, those with single lineage dysplasia have a longer survival and a lower risk of transformation to AML. Thus, RA and RARS with single lineage dysplasia and RA and RARS with multilineage dysplasia appear to be different disease entities.

Therefore, in the refined WHO definition, the RA and RARS categories include only patients with dysplasia limited to the erythroid lineage. For RA and RARS with multilineage dysplasia, a new category was introduced: refractory cytopenia with multilineage dysplasia (RCMD) (*see* Figure 5.7) [8]. In patients with 15% or more ringed sideroblasts, the category is RCMD with ringed sideroblasts (RCMD-RS). It remains unclear if there are important clinical differences between RCMD and RCMD-RS.

New RAEB subgroups
The WHO criteria also further divided the RAEB subgroup into two more specific categories, depending on the number of blasts in the blood and bone marrow: RAEB-1 and RAEB-2 (*see* Figure 5.7) [8]. The RAEB-1 subtype includes patients with 5–9% blasts in the blood and the RAEB-2 subtype includes patients with 10–19% blasts. The distinction is based on data indicating that those with more than 10% blasts have worse outcomes compared to those with fewer blasts [15].

The 5q deletion and 5q– syndrome
Between 16% and 30% of patients with chromosome abnormalities have an interstitial deletion on the long arm of chromosome 5, which represents the most common cytogenetic abnormality in MDS. The deleted region encompasses a 1.5-Mb region that extends between bands 5q31 to 5q32 [40–42]. This is the hypothetical location of a tumor-suppressor gene; however, recent investigations have identified a single allele deletion of the *RPS14* gene as a critical pathogenetic event responsible for the 5q– phenotype [43]. The 5q deletion is associated with a hypoproliferative anemia and dysplastic megakaryocytes in the bone marrow (Figure 5.8). Patients typically have elevated EPO production and red-cell transfusion dependence [40–42].

Within this group of patients is a specific subtype of MDS introduced in the WHO classification: the 5q– syndrome. It is defined by an isolated deletion between bands q21 and q32 on chromosome 5 and characterized by refractory anemia, normal or elevated platelet counts, and megakaryocytes

Figure 5.8 The 5q– syndrome

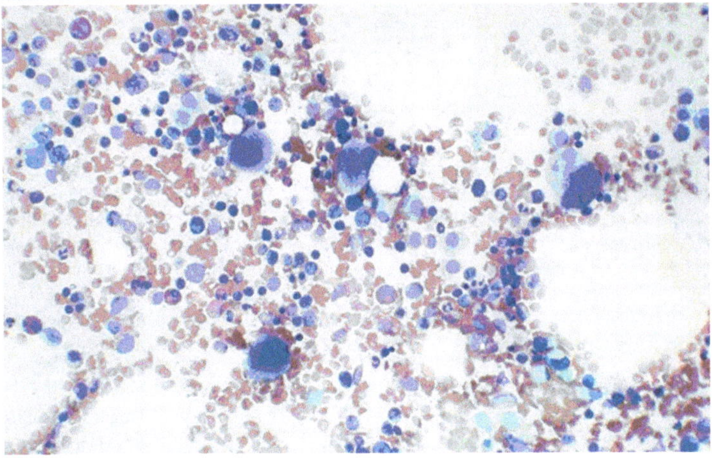

Patients with the 5q– syndrome usually present with refractory macrocytic anemia, normal to increased platelet count, and increased numbers of megakaryocytes, many of which have hypolobated nuclei. The number of blasts in the bone marrow and blood is less than 5%. Reproduced with permission from Chang & Forman [44].

with hypolobated nuclei. Patients must have fewer than 5% blasts in the blood and marrow, and the clinical course is typically indolent [8,41]. This subgroup is now a specifically recognized subtype with specific, targeted therapeutic interventions.

Unclassifiable MDS and CMML

The WHO system also introduced a category for unclassified MDS (MDS-U) [8]. This category includes patients with cytopenias and unilineage dysplasia in granulocytes or megakaryocytes, no or rare blasts in the blood, and less than 5% blasts in the bone marrow (*see* Figure 5.7). Finally, CMML was eliminated from the WHO classification system and recategorized as a disorder with characteristics of both myelodysplasia and myeloproliferation [8].

International Prognostic Scoring System

The IPSS is based on pooled data from seven studies with 816 treatment-naive patients with *de novo* MDS [15]. The scoring system combines clinical, morphologic, and cytogenetic characteristics to predict survival and the risk of AML transformation. To develop the system, a diagnosis of MDS was made using the FAB criteria, and, using a multivariate analysis model, the percentage of bone marrow blasts, karyotype, and the number of cyto-

Figure 5.9 The IPSS system for MDS

Characteristic	Value	Score
Bone marrow blasts (%)	<5	0
	5–10	0.5
	11–20	1.5
	21–30	2.0
Karyotype*	Good	0
	Intermediate	0.5
	Poor	1.0
Cytopenias	0–1	0
	2–3	0.5

Risk group	Sum of score
Low	0
Intermediate-1	0.5–1.0
Intermediate-2	1.5–2.0
High	≥2.5

*Good: diploid, -y, del(5q), del(20q); Poor: chromosome 7 abnormalities or complex (≥3) abnormalities; Intermediate: all others. IPSS, International Prognostic Scoring System. Adapted from Greenberg *et al.* [15].

Figure 5.10 Survival (A) and freedom from AML evolution (B) of MDS patients related to their classification by the IPSS for MDS (Kaplan–Meier curves)

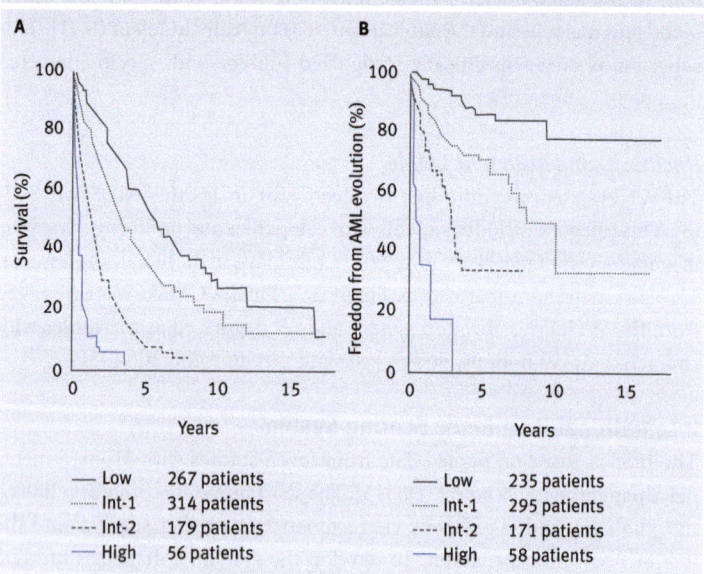

— Low	267 patients
······ Int-1	314 patients
---- Int-2	179 patients
— High	56 patients

— Low	235 patients
······ Int-1	295 patients
---- Int-2	171 patients
— High	58 patients

AML, acute myeloid leukemia; Int, intermediate; IPSS, International Prognostic Scoring System. Reproduced with permission from Greenberg *et al.* [15].

penias were identified as significant independent predictors of survival and AML transformation (Figure 5.9). Age was also determined an important predictor of survival in patients with lower risk disease, and as patient age increased, survival decreased. However, age was not predictive of AML transformation.

To calculate an overall risk score, scores for each independent variable – marrow blast percentage, karyotypes, and number of cytopenias – were generated [15]. These scores were then combined and patients stratified into four risk groups: low, intermediate-1, intermediate-2, and high. Probabilities for survival decreased and AML transformation risk increased with increasing score (Figure 5.10) [15].

The ability of the IPSS to predict survival and AML transformation exceeds that of the FAB by incorporating other disease features (cytogenetics, number of cytopenias), and the tool continues to be an important component in risk stratification and treatment selection in clinical practice [10].

Chapter 6

Management of myelodysplastic syndromes

Multiple management strategies are used for patients with MDS. These strategies range from observation to supportive care for symptom management, to curative therapies such as stem cell transplants with considerable inherent risk.

Current guidelines from the National Comprehensive Cancer Network (NCCN) [10] recommend that treatment strategies be selected based upon several considerations:

International Prognostic Scoring System (IPSS) risk category
- Low risk, intermediate-1 risk, intermediate-2 risk, and high risk.
- Conservative and supportive treatment is generally recommended for low- and intermediate-1-risk patients and more aggressive therapy for those at higher risk.

Patient age and co-morbidities
- These factors determine an individual's ability to tolerate certain treatments.
- High-intensity, high-risk therapeutic options are generally reserved for patients with high-risk disease but who are relatively young and with few co-morbidities.

Relative stability of blood counts over time
- Needed to assess disease progression, transition to AML, and management needs.

Patient preferences

All patients, regardless of risk, should receive appropriate supportive care. Algorithms for treatment strategies according to risk are shown in Figures 6.1 and 6.2. Standardized measures recommended by an International Working Group (IWG) for evaluating response to MDS treatment in clinical trials are shown in Figure 6.3 [45].

Figure 6.1 Algorithm for the treatment of intermediate-2 and high-risk MDS

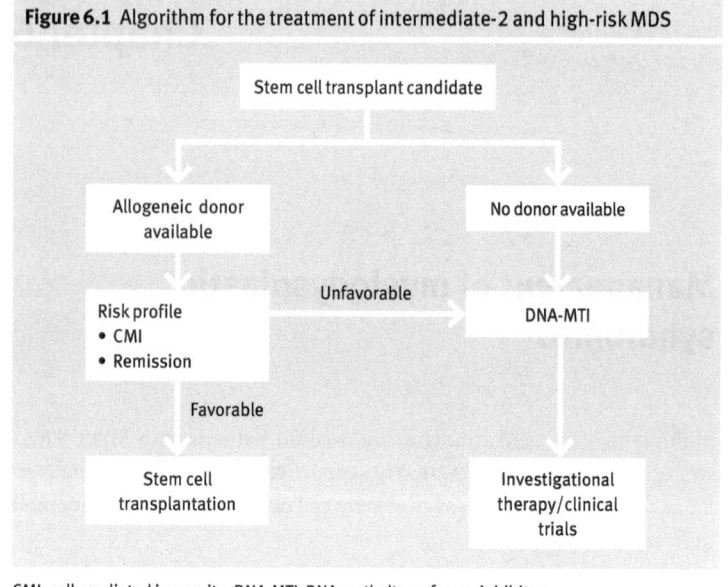

CMI, cell-mediated immunity; DNA-MTI, DNA methyltransferase inhibitor.

Several agents are approved by the FDA for the treatment of MDS, others are recommended by current guidelines, and some are in clinical development. The treatments described in this chapter are those approved by the FDA or recommended by current guidelines.

Supportive care

The symptoms arising from cytopenias associated with MDS can profoundly impact patients' lives. Supportive measures, which are currently considered the standard of care by the community, is aimed at improving QoL [10,46]. Supportive care takes many forms, ranging from clinical monitoring, psychosocial support and QoL assessments to cytokine administration. RBC transfusions are considered for patients with symptomatic anemia and iron chelation with deferoxamine or deferasirox to prevent or reduce transfusion-related iron overload [10]. Platelet transfusions are recommended for patients with severe thrombocytopenia experiencing hemorrhagic complications or at imminent risk for bleeding. Judicious use of antimicrobial agents is imperative for effective management of infections, often accompanied by myeloid growth factors in patients with neutropenia [10,46].

Figure 6.2 Algorithm for the treatment of low- and intermediate-1-risk MDS

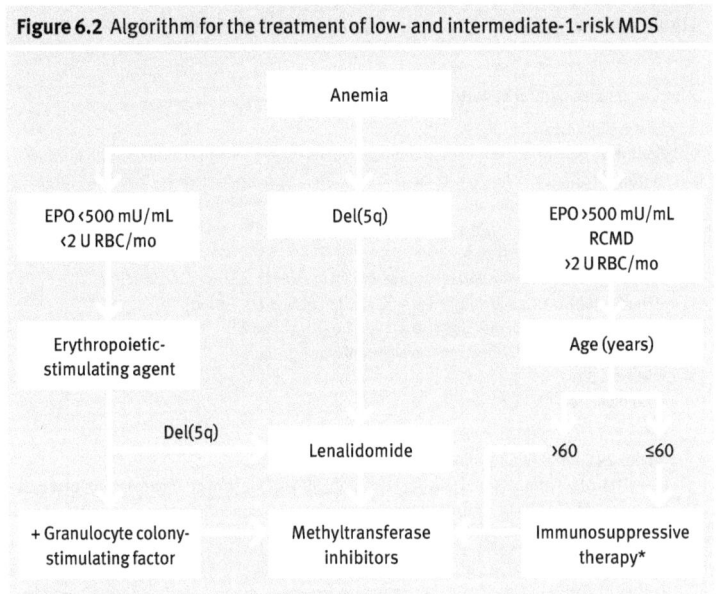

*Consider trisomy 8. EPO, erythropoietin; RCMD, refractory cytopenias with multilineage dysplasia.

Erythropoietic-stimulating agents

Two EPO-stimulating agents (ESAs) are available in the US: epoetin alfa and darbepoetin alfa. Both products are approved by the FDA for the treatment of anemia associated with chronic kidney disease and chemotherapy-associated anemia in nonmyeloid cancers. Neither is specifically indicated for the treatment of MDS-associated anemia.

Nevertheless, both ESAs have been used extensively in the management of MDS-associated anemia [44,47–49]. The restoration of effective erythropoiesis by these agents in responsive patients may provide a sustained rise in hemoglobin and decrease the need for RBC transfusions, thereby decreasing anemia symptoms and improving overall QoL [46]. At least one recent study also suggests that these agents improve patient survival in responding patients [50].

The efficacy of ESAs in clinical trials is measured according to standardized criteria from the IWG, with changes in hemoglobin or transfusion needs as defining variables (*see* Figure 6.3) [45]. A major hemoglobin response is considered an increase from baseline of at least 2 g/dL and elimination of

Figure 6.3 Measurement of response to treatment in myelodysplastic syndromes

Altering disease natural history

1. Complete remission (CR)
   Bone marrow evaluation: Repeat bone marrow showing <5% myeloblasts with normal maturation of all cell lines, with no evidence for dysplasia.* When erythroid precursors constitute <50% of bone marrow nucleated cells, the percentage of blasts is based on all nucleated cells; when there are ≥50% erythroid cells, the percentage blasts should be based on the nonerythroid cells.
   Peripheral blood evaluation (absolute values must last at least 2 months):†
   - Hemoglobin >11 g/dL (untransfused, patient not on erythropoietin)
   - Neutrophils ≥1500/mm³ (not on a myeloid growth factor)
   - Platelets ≥100,000/mm³ (not on a thrombopoetic agent)
   - Blasts, 0%
   - No dysplasia*

2. Partial remission (PR) (absolute values must last at least 2 months)
   All the CR criteria (if abnormal before treatment), except:
   Bone marrow evaluation: Blasts decreased by 50% or more over pretreatment, or a less advanced MDS FAB classification than pretreatment. Cellularity and morphology are not relevant.

3. Stable disease
   Failure to achieve at least a PR, but with no evidence of progression for at least 2 months.

4. Failure
   Death during treatment or disease progression characterized by worsening of cytopenias, increase in the percentage bone marrow blasts, or progression to an MDS FAB subtype more advanced than pretreatment.

5. Relapse after CR or PR – one or more of the following:
   - Return to pretreatment bone marrow blast percentage.
   - Decrement of ≥50% from maximum remission/response levels in granulocytes or platelets.
   - Reduction in hemoglobin concentration by at least 2 g/dL or transfusion dependence.‡

6. Disease progression
   - For patients with <5% blasts: a ≥50% increase in blasts to >5% blasts.
   - For patients with 5–10% blasts: a ≥50% increase to >10% blasts.
   - For patients with 10–20% blasts: a ≥50% increase to >20% blasts.
   - For patients with 20–30% blasts: a ≥50% increase to >30% blasts.
   - One or more of the following: ≥50% decrement from maximum remission/response levels in granulocytes or platelets, reduction in hemoglobin concentration by at least 2 g/dL, or transfusion dependence.‡

7. Disease transformation
   Transformation to AML (≥30% blasts).

8. Survival and progression-free survival

Cytogenic response

(Requires 20 analyzable metaphases using conventional cytogenetic techniques.)
Major: No detectable cytogenetic abnormality, if preexisting abnormality was present.
Minor: ≥50% reduction in abnormal metaphases.
Fluorescent *in situ* hybridization may be used as a supplement to follow a specifically defined cytogenetic abnormality.

Figure 6.3 Continued Measurement of response to treatment in myelodysplastic syndromes

Quality of life

(Measured by an instrument such as the FACT questionnaire.)
Clinically useful improvement in specific domains:
- Physical
- Functional
- Emotional
- Social
- Spiritual

Hematologic improvement (HI)

(Improvements must last at least 2 months in the absence of ongoing cytotoxic therapy.)[†]
HI should be described by the number of individual, positively affected cell lines (e.g., HI-E; HI-E + HI-N; HI-E + HI-P + HI-N).

1. Erythroid response (HI-E)
    Major response: For patients with pretreatment hemoglobin <11 g/dL, >2 g/dL increase in hemoglobin; for RBC transfusion-dependent patients, transfusion independence.
    Minor response: For patients with pretreatment hemoglobin <11 g/dL, 1–2 g/dL increase in hemoglobin; for RBC transfusion-dependent patients, 50% decrease in transfusion requirements.

2. Platelet response (HI-P)
    Major response: For patients with a pretreatment platelet count <100,000/mm³, an absolute increase of 30,000/mm³ or more; for platelet transfusion-dependent patients, stabilization of platelet counts and platelet transfusion independence.
    Minor response: For patients with a pretreatment platelet count <100,000/mm³, a ≥50% increase in platelet count with a net increase >10,000/mm³ but <30,000/mm³.

3. Neutrophil response (HI-N)
    Major response: For absolute neutrophil count (ANC) <1500/mm³ before therapy, at least a 100% increase, or an absolute increase of >500/mm³, whichever is greater.
    Minor response: For ANC <1500/mm³ before therapy, ANC increase of at least 100%, but absolute increase <500/mm³.

4. Progression/relapse after HI
    One or more of the following: a ≥50% decrement from maximum response levels in granulocytes or platelets, a reduction in hemoglobin concentration by at least 2 g/dL, or transfusion dependence.[‡]

For a designated response (CR, PR, HI), all relevant response criteria must be noted on at least two successive determinations at least 1 week apart after an appropriate period following therapy (e.g., 1 month or longer). *The presence of mild megaloblastoid changes may be permitted if they are thought to be consistent with treatment effect. However, persistence of pretreatment abnormalities (e.g., pseudo-Pelger–Hüet cells, ringed sideroblasts, dysplastic megakaryocytes) are not consistent with CR. [†]In some circumstances, protocol therapy may require the initiation of further treatment (e.g., consolidation, maintenance) before the 2-month period. Such patients can be included in the response category into which they fit at the time the therapy is started. [‡]In the absence of another explanation such as acute infection, gastrointestinal bleeding, hemolysis, etc. Reproduced with permission from Cheson *et al.* [45].

transfusion requirements. A minor response is considered an increase in hemoglobin of 1–2 g/dL from baseline or at least a 50% reduction in transfusion requirements [45]. The overall hematologic improvement rate is defined as the sum of the major and minor responses among all lineages.

Epoetin alfa is a glycoprotein that stimulates the division and maturation of committed RBC precursors, thereby increasing RBC production. In multiple series of unselected MDS patients, response rates have ranged from 15% to 25% [47,51]. In a recent meta-analysis, response rates measured according to increases in hemoglobin were 32.1% in single-arm studies and 27.3% when compared with controls in comparative studies [49]. Response rates may be maximized when this product is given specifically to patients with a favorable profile for ESA response characterized by a serum EPO level <500 mU/mL and RBC transfusion needs <2 units/month (Figure 6.4) [10,51].

The addition of a myeloid growth factor, such as granulocyte colony-stimulating factor (G-CSF) or granulocyte-macrophage colony-stimulating factor (GM-CSF), may potentiate responses to epoetin alfa, improve response rates, and improve QoL [46,52,53]. The improved responses may be sustained for many months (Figure 6.5) [54].

Darbepoetin alfa is a longer-acting ESA that is administered at intervals of once-weekly to every 3 weeks. In clinical trials, darbepoetin alfa produced response rates ranging from 45% to 55% in predominantly low-risk and intermediate-1-risk patients [49,55,56]. Treatment-naive patients had higher response rates, with elevations in hemoglobin associated with improved QoL [55,56].

Responses to ESAs typically occur within 6–8 weeks [52,57,58]. If no response is observed, an escalation in dose should be considered, and treatment should be discontinued after 8–12 weeks in patients who remain unresponsive [46]. Epoetin alfa and darbepoetin alfa are generally considered safe and well tolerated, with several studies suggesting that these ESAs improve survival in low-risk and intermediate-1-risk patients that respond to treatment [59–61]. However, in 2007, the FDA issued a safety alert warning that these agents may be associated with an increased risk of death, tumor growth, and thromboembolic events in non-MDS patients treated with dosages targeting hemoglobin levels greater than 12 g/dL [62]. Nevertheless, current guidelines consider these agents a safe and important part of an overall treatment strategy for patients with MDS [10].

Myeloid growth factors

As already mentioned, myeloid growth factors (G-CSF and GM-CSF) may potentiate the effects of epoetin alpha and increase the response rate

Figure 6.4 Model for response prediction with epoetin plus G-CSF therapy in myelodysplastic syndromes

Serum erythropoietin level (U/L)	RBC transfusion requirements
‹100 = add 2 points	‹2 U/mo = add 2 points
100–500 = add 1 point	≥2 U/mo = subtract 2 points
›500 = subtract 3 points	

Total score	Erythroid response*
Good: › +1 point	74% (n=34)
Intermediate: −1 to +1 point	23% (n=31)
Poor: ‹ 1 point	7% (n=39)

*Response was defined as ›1.5 g/dL, hemoglobin increment, or achievement of transfusion independence. G-CSF, granulocyte colony-stimulating factor; RBC, red blood cell. Reproduced with permission from Steensma [46].

Figure 6.5 Response to combined EPO and G-CSF in an 81-year-old female with refractory anemia with ringed sideroblasts previously unresponsive to EPO alone

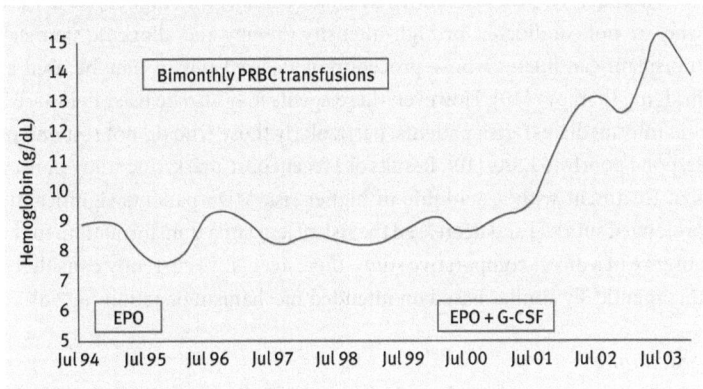

With the continued therapy, response has persisted through March 2006.
EPO, erythropoietin; G-CSF, granulocyte colony-stimulating factor;
PRBC, packed red blood cells. Reproduced with permission from Shadduck
et al. [54].

[46,52–54]. When administered alone to neutropenic patients, these agents increase neutrophil counts. Their impact on survival or disease progression, however, has not been systematically evaluated [63]. Generally, myeloid growth factors should only be given to patients who have an inadequate response to epoetin alfa for the management of anemia, or in conjunction with antibiotics in neutropenic patients with active infection [46].

Platelet growth factors

Thrombopoietin, the native growth factor regulating platelet production, was first cloned in the 1990s, but clinical development was initially halted because of immunogenicity [46,48]. Currently, three thrombopoietic agents are in development: romiplostim (AMG531), AKR-501, and eltrombopag (SB-497115). Multiple clinical trials evaluating romiplostim in MDS are ongoing and preliminary results are encouraging [33,48,64].

DNA methyltransferase inhibitors (epigenetic modification)

The DNA methyltransferase inhibitors, or so-called hypomethylating agents, azacitidine and decitabine, are nucleoside analogs that induce DNA hypomethylation in MDS progenitors, thereby restoring expression of methylation-silenced genes, and re-establishing normal cell differentiation and growth programs. Both agents are specifically approved by the FDA for the treatment of MDS and are considered a low-intensity form of therapy [10].

Candidates for these treatments include patients with higher risk disease who are not candidates for high-intensity therapy and allogenic stem cell transplant candidates whose procedure is delayed (i.e., it may be used as bridging therapy) [10]. However, these agents may also be used in low-risk and intermediate-1-risk patients, particularly those who do not respond or respond poorly to ESAs [10]. Results of a recent post-marketing study showed that treatment with azacitidine in higher risk MDS patients significantly prolonged survival and decreased the risk of leukemia transformation. In the absence of a direct comparative study, these agents are currently considered therapeutically similar based on intended mechanism of action [65,66].

Azacitidine

Azacitidine is an analog of cytidine that has dual effects to (1) disrupt the metabolism of nucleic acid causing direct cytotoxicity, and (2) promote DNA hypomethylation and restore maturation potential. Azacitidine preferentially exerts its cytotoxic effects on actively dividing cells, leaving nonproliferative cells relatively unaffected. It is approved by the FDA for the treatment of all subtypes of MDS (FAB classifications) [67].

In a pivotal phase III trial, 191 *de novo* and secondary MDS patients, stratified according to the FAB classification, were randomized to treatment with azacitidine or standard care (antimicrobial therapy and transfusions) [65]. Azacitidine was administered subcutaneously (75 mg/m^2/day) for 7 days every 4 weeks. If no response was observed after two cycles, the dose was increased by 33% if tolerated. After 4 months, patients in the supportive care arm were permitted to cross over to azacitidine treatment if their disease worsened. Patients were evaluated for complete and partial responses, hematologic improvement, and QoL.

Baseline characteristics between treatment groups were well balanced [65]. IPSS scores were similar, and, overall, 9% of patients were considered low risk, 45% intermediate-1 risk, 27% intermediate-2 risk, and 19% high risk. A total of 60% of azacitidine-treated patients responded to treatment versus 5% of patients in the supportive care only group ($p<0.0001$). Responses to azacitidine included complete response in 7%, partial response in 16%, and 37% were hematologically improved, whereas corresponding results in the supportive care arm were 0%, 0%, and 5%, respectively (p-values versus azacitidine: 0.01, <0.0001, and <0.0001, respectively) [65]. Responses in all three hematopoietic lineages were observed in 23% of azacitidine-treated patients compared to no multilineage improvements in the supportive care arm. Responses occurred across all FAB subgroups.

The median time to AML transformation or death among azacitidine-treated patients was 21 months versus 13 months in patients randomized to supportive care ($p=0.007$). Transformation to AML occurred in 15% of azacitidine-treated patients compared to a frequency of 38% in the supportive arm ($p=0.001$) (Figure 6.6) [65]. Azacitidine treatment also yielded a greater improvement in QoL measures of fatigue ($p=0.001$); physical functioning ($p=0.002$); dyspnea ($p=0.0014$); psychosocial distress ($p=0.015$); and positive affect ($p=0.0077$).

These findings were recently updated in a reanalysis of three previously reported trials, which retrospectively applied the IPSS and evaluated responses according to the IWG 2000 criteria (*see* Figure 6.3) [68]. The analysis reported IWG complete remission rates ranging from 10% to 17% in the three trials, and hematologic improvement rates ranging from 23% to 36%.

A second phase III trial (AZA-001) was performed to comply with FDA approval requirements that compared treatment with azacitidine to three conventional care strategies of supportive care alone, low-dose cytarabine, or standard AML induction and consolidation therapy in higher risk MDS patients with IPSS intermediate-2- or high-risk MDS [69]. Median survival was significantly prolonged with azacitidine treatment compared with conventional care (24.4 months versus 15 months; $p=0.0001$), with nearly a doubling of survival at 2 years (50.8% versus 26.2%, respectively). Moreover, azacitidine treatment improved survival compared to conventional care regimens in all prognostic subgroups analyzed, with the greatest improvement observed in patients with poor-risk karyotypes involving chromosome 7. Azacitidine significantly prolonged the median time to AML or death

Figure 6.6 Time to AML transformation or death

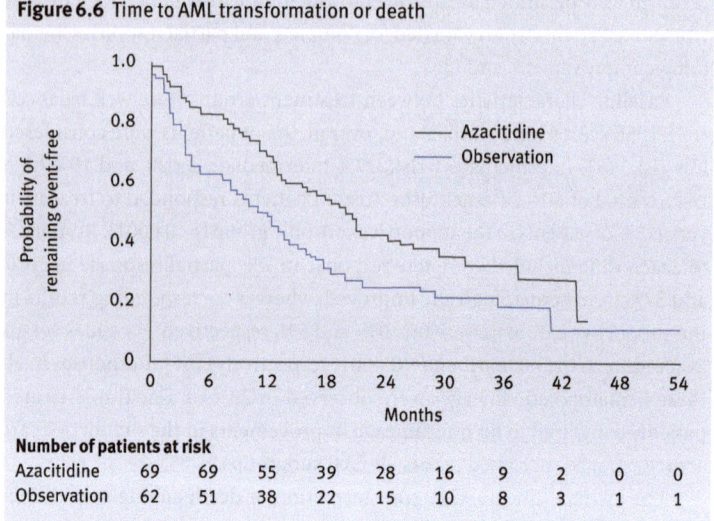

Time was measured from entry on study to the time of first event, either transformation to AML or death, and estimated according to the Kaplan–Meier method. Reproduced with permission from Silverman *et al.* [65].

(13 months vs. 7.6 months; $p=0.003$), and 45% of transfusion-dependent patients treated with azacitidine became transfusion free compared to 11% receiving conventional care [69]. The overall frequency of complete or partial response was 29% for the azacitidine arm compared to 12% for conventional care ($p=0.0001$). Major and minor hematologic improvement according to IWG 2000 criteria occurred in 49% of patients treated with azacitidine compared to 29% of those on the conventional care arm ($p<0.0001$). Hematologic toxicities were comparable for the azacitidine and conventional care arms. This study is the first and only trial in MDS to show a survival advantage with any management strategy for MDS.

A randomized phase II trial investigated alternative dose and schedules of azacitidine in an effort to explore alternatives to the need for weekend treatment with the FDA-approved treatment schedule. Three dose schedules were compared: azacitidine 75 mg/m²/day for 5 days followed by the weekend off and 2 days of treatment (i.e., 5–2–2); azacitidine 50 mg/m²/day for 5 days followed by another 5 days of treatment after a weekend hiatus (5–2–5); and azacitidine 75 mg/m²/day for 5 consecutive days [70]. The primary endpoint of the trial was hematologic improvement using IWG 2000 criteria, with no planned bone marrow evaluations. There was no discernable difference in response rate between the three regimens. Hematologic improvement rates ranged from 44% to 56% with major hematologic improvements occurring in all hematopoietic lineages: erythroid, 33–39%; platelets, 18–22%; and neutrophils, 7–8%. The frequency of transfusion independence was comparable and ranged from 54% to 67%. There was a trend favoring a lower frequency of grade 3 and 4 hematologic toxicity in the patients treated with the 5-day regimen. Among lower-risk patients for whom hematologic improvement is the primary endpoint, these results support utilization of the 5-day schedule of azacitidine administration that preserves hematologic response with potentially less myelosuppression.

Decitabine

Decitabine is a 2′-deoxycytidine analog that, like azacitidine, exerts both an antineoplastic effect after phosphorylation and incorporation into DNA, and acts as a DNA methyltransferase inhibitor to promote hypomethylation. Decitabine is specifically indicated for the treatment of primary and secondary MDS, including all FAB subtypes and intermediate-1-, -2- and high-risk IPSS categories [71]. The recommended dosage is 15 mg/m² administered over 3 hours every 8 hours for 3 days for a cumulative dose of 135 mg/m².

In three phase II trials, which collectively enrolled 180 patients with intermediate- and high-risk MDS, overall response rates in an intention-to-treat analysis were 45%, 26%, and 26%, respectively, and median durations of response of 217 days, 250 days, and 146 days, respectively [72].

In another phase II trial analysis, investigators evaluated the effects of decitabine on platelet response in 162 patients with intermediate-1 or higher risk disease, 126 of whom had thrombocytopenia at the start of treatment [73]. After one cycle of therapy, 58% of thrombocytopenic patients experienced a platelet improvement, with 69% of patients achieving an IWG platelet response with continued treatment that was associated with a longer overall survival. Transient myelosuppression is the most common side effect [72–74].

The phase III registration study compared decitabine and supportive care with supportive care alone in 170 patients with MDS of all FAB subtypes and an IPSS risk score of 0.5 or greater (intermediate-1 risk or higher) [66]. Standard care included RBC and platelet transfusions and myeloid growth factors. Decitabine was administered at a dose of 15 mg/m² as an intravenous infusion over 3 hours every 8 hours for 3 days every 6 weeks for no more than six cycles. QoL was assessed at baseline, at the end of each treatment cycle, and at the end of treatment. The co-primary endpoints included complete and partial response rate according to IWG 2000 criteria and the time to

AML transformation or death. Responses were evaluated using the IWG 2000 criteria (*see* Figure 6.3). Median patient age in the trial was 70 years, approximately 70% of patients had an IPSS score of intermediate-2 or high risk, 71% were dependent on RBC transfusions, and 23% were dependent on platelet transfusions.

The overall complete (9%) plus partial (8%) response rate was 17% in the decitabine arm and 0% in the supportive care arm ($p<0.001$) [66], with responses maintained for a median of 10.3 months. Erythroid hematologic improvement was observed in 13% of decitabine-treated patients versus 7% of patients who received supportive care alone, representing an overall improvement rate (CR + PR + HI) of 30% versus 7%, respectively ($p<0.001$). Responses were similar across subgroups and risk categories.

There was a nonsignificant trend favoring decitabine treatment in the time to AML transformation or death (12.1 versus 7.8 months, $p=0.16$) [66]. However, in patients with intermediate-2 or higher risk MDS, the decitabine effect reached statistical significance (Figure 6.7). QoL was also improved with decitabine, with sustainable improvements observed in global health status, fatigue, and dyspnea ($p<0.05$). Decitabine was well tolerated, with side effects comparable to those observed in the standard care arm.

In an effort to optimize outpatient treatment with decitabine, a lower cumulative dose of decitabine (100 mg/m^2) was investigated in three different administration schedules in patients with advanced MDS or CMML: 20 mg/m^2 intravenous daily for 5 days; 20 mg/m^2 subcutaneously daily for 5 days; and 10 mg/m^2 intravenously daily for 10 days [66]. Complete response rates were 34% versus 21% versus 24%, respectively ($p<0.05$). Research into this off-label dosing regimen is continuing.

Immunomodifying therapy

Immunomodifying therapies comprise a varied group of nonchemotherapy, low-intensity treatments for MDS. These agents include immunosuppressive therapy (IST) such as ATG and cyclosporine A, and immune-potentiating agents such as thalidomide and lenalidomide. These agents have primary or secondary effects on immune abnormalities in patients with MDS, such as decreased natural killer cell activity, antibody-dependent cell killing, mitogenic response, decreased CD4 cells [9], and clonal amplification of hematopoietic-inhibitory T lymphocytes [64].

Response rates to IST are variable [64]; however, those patients whose disease may be most responsive can be characterized by clinical and disease-specific features. In a univariate analysis of the National Institutes of Health (NIH) ATG trial experience, patients less than 60 years of age, those with

Figure 6.7 Patient survival: decitabine versus supportive care

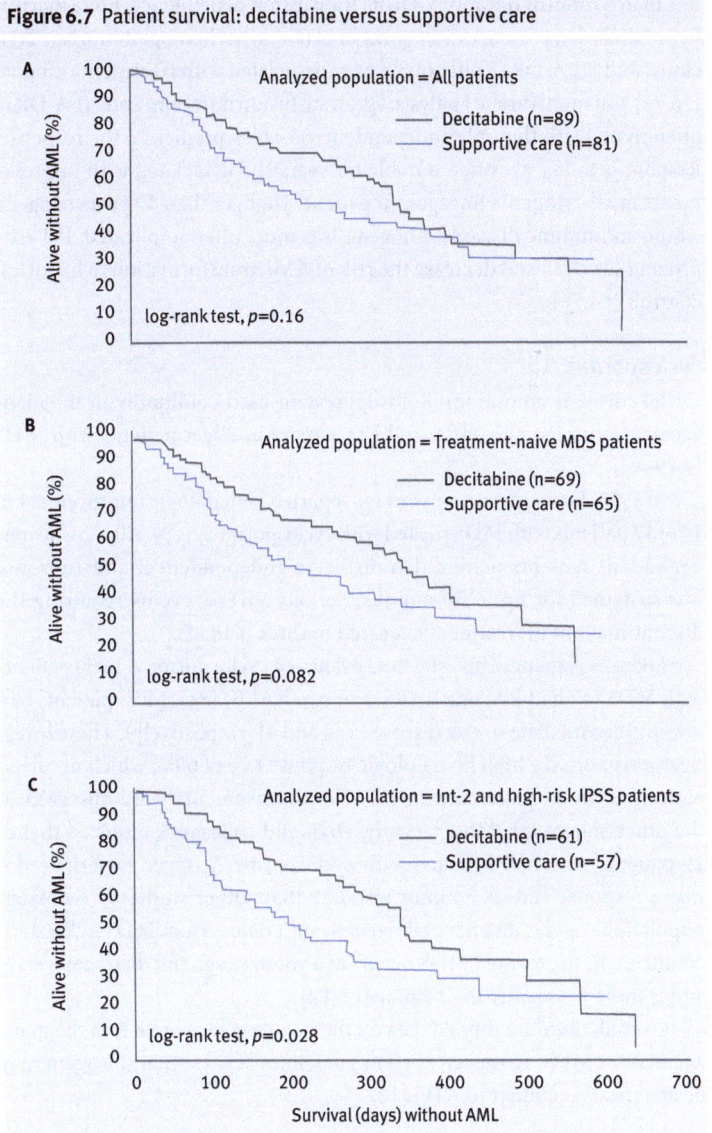

(A) Patients treated with decitabine had a median time to acute myelogenous leukemia (AML) or death that was 4.3 months greater than that noted for patients receiving supportive care alone. (B) Similar improved times to AML or death were observed among patients who were chemotherapy naive or (C) had an International Prognostic Scoring System (IPSS) score of intermediate-2 (Int-2) or higher. Reproduced with permission from Kantarjian *et al.* [66].

less than 6 months duration of RBC transfusion dependence, bone marrow hypocellularity, presence of a paroxysmal nocturnal hemoglobinuria (PNH) clone, and HLA-DR15 phenotype were associated with treatment response [76,77]. On multivariate analysis, age, transfusion duration, and HLA-DR15 phenotype were the only independent variables predictive for response. Responses to IST are often durable for years and associated with improvements in all cytopenia lineages. In patients younger than 60 years of age in whom an immune disease pathogenesis is more often implicated, IST may prolong survival, and decrease the risk of AML transformation to historical controls [64,78].

Cyclosporine

Cyclosporine is an oral immunosuppressant used commonly in the management of organ allografts, and has activity in select patients with MDS [9,79–82].

In 1998, Jonásova and co-workers reported hematologic improvement in 14 of 17 patients with MDS treated with cyclosporine A [79]. All transfusion-dependent patients achieved transfusion independence, and response was sustained for up to 30 months. Serious adverse events requiring the discontinuation of treatment occurred in three patients.

Likewise, Japanese investigators evaluated cyclosporine A in 50 patients with MDS (47 had RA, one RARS, and two RAEB) [81]. Most patients had low- or intermediate-1-risk disease (n=4 and 41, respectively). These investigators reported a high hematologic response rate of 60%, which occurred entirely in those patients with RA. No improvements were observed in the other subgroups. Most recently, Dixit and colleagues reported that of 19 patients with MDS treated with cyclosporine A, seven experienced a major response and six a minor response [83]. Other studies in the Asian population suggest distinct pathogenetic differences from MDS in Western countries: in the former, MDS occurs at a younger age (median, <60 years) and is more frequently IST responsive [84].

Overall, there are limited data on the use of cyclosporine A in the management of MDS. However, current guidelines suggest that the agent may be an effective adjunct to ATG [10].

Antithymocyte globulin

ATG is a lymphocyte-selective horse- or rabbit-derived serotherapy that selectively depletes thymus-dependent lymphocytes. It is approved by the FDA for the management of allograft rejection in renal transplant patients and aplastic anemia [85]. The overlapping biology of aplastic anemia and MDS served as the rationale for the investigation of ATG in MDS [9,86–89].

Molldrem and co-workers at the NIH treated 61 RBC transfusion-dependent patients with equine ATG at 40 mg/kg/day for 4 days [90]. RBC transfusion independence was achieved by 34% of patients within a median of 8 months of treatment. Transfusion independence was maintained for a median of 32 months. Of the 41 patients with severe thrombocytopenia, 56% experienced platelet increases ranging from 25,000 to 290,000/μL. Actuarial survival at 34 months was 64% [90]. Additional NIH experience suggests that the combination of ATG with cyclosporine A may have superior activity in MDS, similar to its effect in aplastic anemia [86,91].

Thalidomide and lenalidomide

Thalidomide and its structural derivative lenalidomide are members of a proprietary class of agents referred to as immunomodulatory drugs or IMiDs. Both agents possess a broad capacity to modify ligand-activated receptor signals that results in antiangiogenic effects, inhibition of TNF-α and other inflammatory cytokine elaboration, in addition to immune-potentiating effects [64,92,93].

In one of the initial studies of thalidomide in MDS, Raza and colleagues reported promising response rates, but excess neurosedative toxicity [94]. The study enrolled 83 patients with thalidomide administered at an initial dosage of 100 mg/day, which was increased to 400 mg/day, as tolerated. In the intention-to-treat analysis, 19% of patients had hematologic improvement. No complete responses were noted, but among the 16 responders, 15 had an erythroid response and one patient had a major platelet response. Subsequent studies evaluated doses ranging from 200 to 1000 mg/day in lower and higher risk patients, and reported variable rates of hematologic improvement or partial responses ranging from 20% to 60% [95–97].

Despite encouraging activity, cumulative and dose-dependent toxicity limits thalidomide therapy in this generally elderly disease population. In Raza and coworker's trial, 32 of the 83 patients enrolled could not complete the 12-week study period, with 14 of these patients withdrawing because of treatment-related toxicity [94]. The most common adverse effects were fatigue, constipation, dyspnea, fluid retention, dizziness, rash, peripheral neuropathy, fever, headache, and nausea [64,94].

Lenalidomide, which has a 100- to 1000-fold greater *in vitro* potency than thalidomide, displayed less toxicity in clinical studies. In MDS clinical trials, lenalidomide has shown remarkable efficacy, particularly in patients with an interstitial deletion of chromosome 5q with a manageable toxicity profile (Figure 6.8) [41,64,98,99]. Lenalidomide is approved by the FDA for the treatment of patients with transfusion-dependent anemia due to low- or intermediate-1-risk MDS associated with the deletion of chromosome 5q [100].

The initial dose-finding study of lenalidomide enrolled 43 patients with symptomatic or transfusion-dependent anemia with a FAB diagnosis of MDS [98]. Three oral dosing schedules: 25 mg/day, 10 mg/day, and 10 mg/day for 21 days every 4 weeks were investigated. Hematologic responses were evaluated according to the IWG 2000 criteria (see Figure 6.3).

The majority of patients (77%) had either RA (RA, 47%) or RARS (30%) with low- or intermediate-1-risk disease in 86% of patients. Major erythroid responses were observed in 49% of patients and minor responses in 7% for an overall erythroid response rate of 56% [98]. Of the 32 patients who were RBC transfusion-dependent at enrollment, 20 (65%) achieved transfusion independence. Hematologic response rate varied by disease karyotype with 83% of patients with the 5q31 deletion (n=12) responding, compared with a response rate of 57% patients with a normal karyotype, and 12% among those with other cytogenetic abnormalities. Remarkably, lenalidomide reversed dysplastic features in bone marrow specimens in patients with 5q deletion that experienced cytogenetic improvement (Figure 6.9).

Lenalidomide lacked the neurotoxicity that plagued thalidomide [98]. Thrombocytopenia and neutropenia were the most common and dose-related adverse events, occurring in 74% and 28% of patients, respectively. Myelosuppression resulted in the interruption of treatment in 77% of patients

Figure 6.8 Comparison of erythroid and cytogenetic responses in patients with and without 5q deletion treated with lenalidomide

	Study 1		Study 2	Study 3	
	del(5q) (n=12)	No del(5q) (n=43)	No del(5q) (n=215)	del(5q) only (n=111)	del(5q) + other abnormalities (n=37)
Erythroid response, major + minor (%)	83	45	43	69	49
Major response or transfusion independence (%)	73	42	26	72	54
Major cytogenic response (%)	83	12	19	77	62
Complete cytogenic response (%)	75	12	8	45	43

Reproduced with permission from Melchert & List [64].

Figure 6.9 Morphologic changes in a bone marrow specimen from a patient with a 5q31.1 deletion

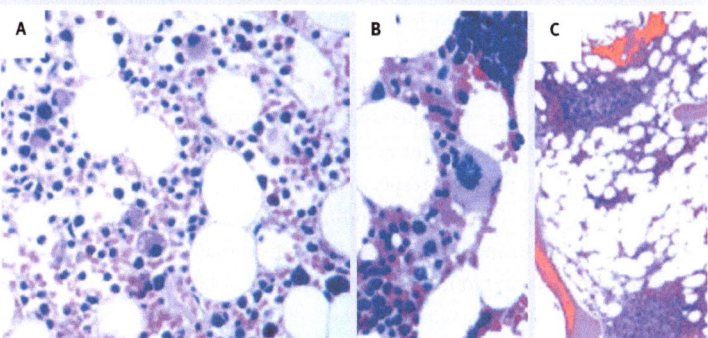

Numerous small, mononuclear megakaryocytes are readily identified in the bone marrow specimen obtained by trephine biopsy before treatment (A; hematoxylin and eosin). After 16 weeks of lenalidomide therapy, megakaryocytes appear normal in size and have multiple nuclei (B; hematoxylin and eosin), and multiple aggregates of benign-appearing lymphocytes are apparent (C; hematoxylin and eosin). Reproduced with permission from List *et al.* [98].

receiving the 25-mg dose after a median 4.6 weeks of treatment versus 62% in those receiving 10 mg/day (median 8.5 weeks), and 47% in those patients who received 10 mg/day for 21 days (median 6 weeks). Treatment was resumed after a median of 22 days. Pruritus, which was generally transient and limited to the scalp, was reported by 28% of patients. Other adverse events included diarrhea (21%) and urticaria (14%) [98].

These findings were confirmed in subsequent multicenter phase II studies [98,99]. The FDA registration trial involved 148 patients with 5q– MDS treated with 10 mg lenalidomide given for 21 days every 4 weeks or daily. Eligibility was restricted to patients with low- or intermediate-1-risk disease with transfusion-dependent anemia and a chromosome 5q deletion either alone or with additional cytogenetic abnormalities. The primary endpoint of the trial was the proportion of patients achieving transfusion-independence with a 1 g/dL or greater rise in hemoglobin for 8 weeks or longer. Secondary endpoints included the duration of transfusion independence, minor erythroid response, cytogenetic, and pathological responses, and safety.

Median age was 71 years and 66% of patients were women [98]. FAB subtypes included RA (52%), RAEB (20%), and RARS (12%).

Overall, 76% of patients responded to treatment. Transfusion independence was achieved by 99 (67%) patients and 13 patients had a 50% or more reduction in the number of needed transfusions after 24 weeks of lenalidomide treatment [98]. Median duration of transfusion-independence exceeded 2 years. Age, gender, FAB and IPSS categories, and cytogenetic pattern did not influence response rates. Cytogenetic analysis was performed in 85 patients, of which 45% achieved a complete cytogenetic response (i.e., remission) after 24 weeks of treatment and 28% achieved a partial response.

Lenalidomide was well tolerated with manageable myelosuppressive effects [98]. Moderate-to-severe neutropenia and thrombocytopenia occurred in 55% and 44% of patients, respectively. There were 11 deaths during the extended treatment follow-up, including three possible treatment-related deaths due to neutropenic-associated infection that occurred early after study activation owing to insufficient frequency of laboratory monitoring. Dosage adjustments were required in 84% of patients, the majority of which occurred during the first 8 weeks of lenalidomide treatment. Only 32% of patients continued to receive 10 mg/day, and 30 patients (20%) discontinued treatment early because of adverse events.

Hematopoietic stem cell transplantation

HSCT is a high-intensity and potentially curative therapy. Allogeneic HSCT from HLA-matched sibling donors yields long-term disease-free survival rates in 30–50% of patients [101,102]. Wide utilization of HSCT, however, is also limited by associated morbidities such as mucositis, graft versus host disease (GVHD), veno-occlusive disease, transplantation-related lung injury, infection, and high mortality. HSCT-related mortality rate ranges from 30% to 50% [18,101,102]. Moreover, only approximately one-third of patients may have an HLA-identical sibling donor [103]. Therefore, although this procedure is potentially curative, it is reserved for high functioning, younger patients (less than 60 years) with higher-risk disease [9,10,18,104].

Stem cell transplants from HLA genotypically matched, unrelated donor HSCTs are now yielding comparable success rates in MDS patients, but remain age-restricted [9]. Indeed, in a review of 510 patients with MDS who received marrow transplants from unrelated donors, the probability of disease-free survival at 2 and 4 years post-transplantation was 29% and 26%, respectively [103]. Acute GVHD grades II to IV occurred in 47% of patients and the treatment-related mortality was high (54%) [103]. New lower intensity conditioning regimens offer the prospect of lower procedure-related morbidity and mortality.

Intensive chemotherapy

Given the powerful disease-modifying effect of azacitidine in the AZA-001 phase III trial, intensive chemotherapy should be reserved for investigational studies and considered perhaps only for high-intensity therapy candidates with favorable or intermediate risk karyotypes or who require a reduction in the marrow leukemia burden prior to transplantation [10]. However, as with HSCT, there is a much higher attendant morbidity and mortality compared to hypomethylating agents, and the NCCN guidelines therefore recommend that these treatments be given in the context of a clinical trial [10].

References

1. Cortes JE, List A, Kantarjian H. Myelodysplastic syndromes. In: Cancer Management: A Multidisciplinary Approach, 10th Edition. Edited by R Pazdur, LR Coia, WJ Hoskins, et al. CMP Medica 2007–2008.
2. Heaney ML, Golde DW. Myelodysplasia. N Engl J Med 1999; 340:1649–1660.
3. Sekeres MA, List A. Immunomodulation in myelodysplastic syndromes. Best Pract Res Clin Haematol 2006; 19:757–767.
4. Kantarjian H, Giles F, List A, et al. The incidence and impact of thrombocytopenia in myelodysplastic syndromes. Cancer 2007; 109:1705–1714.
5. Girtovitis FI, Ntaios G, Papdopoulos A, et al. Defective platelet aggregation in myelodysplastic syndromes. Acta Haematol 2007; 118:117–122.
6. List AF, Sandberg AA, Doll DC. Chapter 83: Myelodysplastic syndromes. In: Wintrobe's Clinical Hematology. Volume 2, 11th edition. Edited by JP Greer, J Foerster, JN Lukens, et al. Lippincott Williams & Wilkins, 2004.
7. Bennett JM, Catovsky D, Daniel MT, et al. Proposals for the classification of the myelodysplastic syndromes. Br J Haematol 1982 51:189–199.
8. Vardiman JW, Harris NL, Brunning RD. The World Health Organization (WHO) classification of the myeloid neoplasms. Blood 2002; 100:2292–2302.
9. Greenberg PL, Young NS, Gattermann N. Myelodysplastic syndromes. Hematol Am Soc Hematol Educ Program 2002:136–161.
10. National Comprehensive Cancer Network (NCCN). NCCN Clinical Practice Guidelines in Oncology. Myelodysplastic Syndromes. V.2.2008. Available at: www.nccn.org/ professionals/physician_gls/PDF/mds.pdf. Last accessed February 12, 2008.
11. Ma X, Does M, Raza A, et al. Myelodysplastic syndromes. Incidence and survival in the United States. Cancer 2007; 109:1536–1542.
12. Paul B, Reid MM, Davison EV, et al. Familial myelodysplasia: progressive disease associated with emergence of monosomy 7. Br J Haematol 1987; 65:321–323.
13. Maserati E, Minelli A, Menna G, et al. Familial myelodysplastic syndromes, monosomy 7/ trisomy 8, and mutator effects. Cancer Genet Cytogenet 2004; 148:155–158.
14. Nisse C, Haguenoer JM, Grandbastien B, et al. Occupational and environmental risk factors of the myelodysplastic syndromes in the North of France. Br J Haematol 2001; 112:927–935.
15. Greenberg P, Cox C, LeBeau MM, et al. International scoring system for evaluating prognosis in myelodysplastic syndromes. Blood 1997; 89:2079–2088.
16. Pomeroy C, Oken MM, Rydell RE, et al. Infection in the myelodysplastic syndromes. Am J Med 1991; 90:338–344.
17. Estey E. Acute myeloid leukemia and myelodysplastic syndromes in older patients. J Clin Oncol 2007; 10:1908–1915.

18. Sekeres M, List A. Alternative treatments for myelodysplastic syndromes. Semin Hematol 2005; 42:S32–S37.

19. Rajapaksa R, Ginzton N, Rott LS, et al. Altered oncoprotein expression and apoptosis in myelodysplastic syndrome marrow cells. Blood 1996; 88:4275–4287.

20. Allampallam K, Shetty V, Mundle S, et al. Biological significance of proliferation, apoptosis, cytokines and monocyte/macrophage cells in bone marrow biopsies of 145 patients with myelodysplastic syndrome. Int J Hematol 2002; 75:289–297.

21. Hirai H. Molecular mechanisms of myelodysplastic syndrome. Jpn J Clin Oncol 2003; 33:153–160.

22. Davis RE, Greenberg PL. Bcl-2 expression by myeloid precursors in myelodysplastic syndromes: relation to disease progression. Leuk Res 1998; 22:767–777.

23. Quesnel B, Guillerm G, Vereecque R, et al. Methylation of the p15INK4b gene in myelodysplasic syndromes is frequent and acquired during disease progression. Blood 1998; 91:2985–2990.

24. Jansen AJG, Essink-Bot ML, Beckers EAM, et al. Quality of life measurement in patients with transfusion-dependent myelodysplastic syndromes. Br J Haematol 2003; 121:270–274.

25. Steensma DP, Heptinstall KV, Johnson VM, et al. Common troublesome symptoms and their impact on quality of life in patients with myelodysplastic syndromes (MDS): Results of a large internet-based survey. Leuk Res 2008; 32:691–698.

26. Pomeroy C, Oken MM, Rydell RE, et al. Infection in the myelodysplastic syndromes. Am J Med 1991; 90:338–344.

27. Mele L, Ricci P, Nosari A, et al. Invasive fungal infection in patients with myelodysplastic syndrome: a report of twelve cases. Leuk Lymphoma 2002; 43:1613–1617.

28. Salacz ME, Lankiewicz MW, Weissman DE. Management of thrombocytopenia in bone marrow failure: A review. J Palliative Med 2007; 10:236–244.

29. Cohen P. Sweet's syndrome: a neutrophilic dermatosis classically associated with acute onset and fever. Clin Dermatol 2000; 18:265–282.

30. Vignon-Pennamen MD, Juillard C, Rybojad M. Chronic recurrent lymphocytic sweet syndrome as a predictive marker of myelodysplasia a report of 9 cases. Arch Dermatol 2006; 142:1170–1176.

31. List FA, Gonzalez-Osete G, Kummet T, et al. Granulocytic sarcoma in myelodysplastic syndromes: clinical marker of disease acceleration. Am J Med 1991; 90:274–276.

32. Cohen PR. Sweet's syndrome – a comprehensive review of an acute febrile neutrophilic dermatosis. Orphanet J Rare Dis 2007; 2:34.

33. Sadick N, Edlin D, Myskowski PL, et al. Granulocytic sarcoma. A new finding in the setting of preleukemia. Arch Dermatol 1984; 120:1341–1343.

34. Stenchever MA, Goff B (Eds). Atlas of Clinical Gynecology: Gynecologic Pathology. Philadelphia, PA; Current Medicine Group, 1998.

35. Kezuka T, Usui N, Suzuki E, et al. Ocular complications in myelodysplastic syndromes as preleukemic disorders. Jpn J Ophthalmol 2005; 49:377–383.

36. Sobecks R, Theil K. Atlas of Cancer. Edited by M Markman, M Kalaycio. Philadelphia, PA; Current Medicine Group LLC, 2002.

37. Michaux JL, Martiat P. Chronic myelomonocytic leukemia (CMML) — a myelodysplastic or myeloproliferative syndrome? Leuk Lymphoma 1993; 9:35–41.

38. Germing U, Gattermann N, Aivado M, et al. Two types of acquired idiopathic sideroblastic anaemia (AISA): a time-tested distinction. Br J Haematol 2000; 108:724–728.

39. Germing U, Gattermann N, Strupp C, et al. Validation of the WHO proposals for a new classification of primary myelodysplastic syndromes: a retrospective analysis of 1600 patients. Leuk Res 2000; 24:983–999.

40. Giagounidis AA, Germing U, Haase S, et al. Clinical, morphological, cytogenetic, and prognostic features of patients with myelodysplastic syndromes and del(5q) including band q31. Leukemia 2004; 18:113–1139.

41. List A, Dewald G, Bennett J, et al. Lenalidomide in the myelodysplastic syndrome with chromosome 5q deletion. N Engl J Med 2006; 355:1456–1465.

42. Bernasconi P, Klersy C, Boni M, et al. Incidence and prognostic significance of karyotype abnormalities in de novo primary myelodysplastic syndromes: a study on 331 patients from a single institution. Leukemia 2005; 19:1424–1431.

43. Ebert BL, Pretz J, Bosco J, et al. Identification of RPS14 as a 5q- syndrome gene by RNA interference screen. Nature 2008; 451:335–339.

44. Chang K, Forman S. Atlas of Clinical Hematology. Edited by JO Armitage. Philadelphia, PA; Current Medicine Group LLC, 2004.

45. Cheson BD, Bennett JM, Kantarjian H, et al. Report of an international working group to standardize response criteria for myelodysplastic syndromes. Blood 2000; 96:3671–3674.

46. Steensma DP. Risk-based management of myelodysplastic syndrome. Oncology 2007; 21:43–54.

47. Stein RS, Abels RI, Krantz SB. Pharmacologic doses of recombinant human erythropoietin in the treatment of myelodysplastic syndromes. Blood 1991; 78:1658–1663.

48. Hellström-Lindberg E, Malcovati L. Support care and use of hematopoietic growth factors in myelodysplastic syndromes. Sem Hematol 2008; 45:14–22.

49. Ross SD, Allen IE, Probst CA, et al. Efficacy and safety of erythropoieses-stimulating proteins in myelodysplastic syndrome: a systemic review and meta-analysis. Oncologist 2007; 12:1264–1273.

50. Park S, Grabar S, Kelaidi C, et al. Predictive factors of response and survival in myelodysplastic syndrome treated with erythropoietin and G-CSF: the GFM experience. Blood 2008; 111:574–582.

51. Hellström-Lindberg E, Gulbrandesen N, Lindberg G, et al. A validated decision model for treating the anaemia of myelodysplastic syndromes with erythropoietin + granulocyte colony-stimulating factor: significant effects on quality of life. Br J Haematol 2003; 120:1037–1046.

52. Casadevall N, Durieux P, Dubois S, et al. Health, economic, and quality-of-life effects of erythropoietin and granulocyte colony-stimulating factor for the treatment of myelodysplastic syndromes: a randomized, controlled trial. Blood 2004; 104:321–327.

53. Balleari E, Rossi E, Clavio M, et al. Erythropoietin plus granulocyte colony-stimulating factor is better than erythropoietin alone to treat anemia in low-risk myelodysplastic syndromes: results from a randomized single-centre study. Ann Hematol 2006; 85:174–180.

54. Shadduck RK, Latsko JM, Rossetti JM, et al. Recent advances in myelodysplastic syndromes. Exper Hematol 2007; 35:137–143.

55. Stasi R, Abruzzese E, Lanzetta G, et al. Darbepoetin alfa for the treatment of anemic patients with low- and intermediate-1-risk myelodysplastic syndromes. Ann Oncol 2005; 16:1921–1927.

56. Giraldo P, Nomdedeu B, Loscertales J, et al. Darbepoetin for the treatment of anemia in patients with myelodysplastic syndromes. Cancer 2006; 107:2807–2816.

57. Hellström-Lindberg E, Negrin R, Stein R, et al. Erythroid response to treatment with G-CSF plus erythropoietin for the anaemia of patients with myelodysplastic syndromes: proposal for a predictive model. Br J Haematol 1997; 99:344–351.

58. Spiriti MA, Latagliata R, Niscola P, et al. Impact of a new dosing regimen of epoetin alfa on quality of life and anemia in patients with low-risk myelodysplastic syndrome. Ann Hematol 2005; 84:167–176.

59. Jadersten M, Malcovati L, Dybedal L, et al. Treatment with Epo and GCSF improves survival in MDS patients with low transfusion need. Blood [ASH meeting abstract] 2006; 108:158a.

60. Jadersten M, Montgomery SM, Dybeal I, et al. Long-term outcome of treatment of anemia in MDS with erythropoietin and G-CSF. Blood 2005; 106:803–811.

61. Park S, Grabar S, Kelaidi C, et al. Has treatment with EPO +/- G-CSF an impact on progression to AML and survival in low/int-1 risk MDS? A comparison between French-EPO patients with the IMRAW database. Leuk Res 2007; 31(Suppl 1):S113.

62. US Food and Drug Administration. FDA Public Health Advisory Erythropoiesis-Stimulating Agents (ESAs). Available at: www.fda.gov/cder/drug/advisory/RHE2007.htm. Last accessed February 19, 2008.

63. Clavio M, Balleari E, Garrone A, et al. Haemopoietic growth factors in myelodysplastic syndromes: Towards patient-oriented therapy? J Exp Clin Cancer Res 2005; 24:5–16.

64. Melchert M, List A. Targeted therapies in myelodysplastic syndrome. Sem Hematol 2008; 45:31–38.

65. Silverman LR, Demakos EP, Peterson BL, et al. Randomized controlled trial of azacytidine in patients with the myelodysplastic syndrome: a study of the Cancer and Leukemia Group B. J Clin Oncol 2002; 20:2429–2440.

66. Kantarjian H, Issa JJ, Rosenfeld CS, et al. Decitabine improves patient outcomes in myelodysplastic syndromes. Results of a phase III randomized study. Cancer 2006; 106:1794–1803.

67. Vidaza® (azacytidine for injection) prescribing information, January 2007. Available at: www.vidaza.com/download/download.ashx?download=1. Last accessed February 20, 2008.

68. Silverman LR, McKenzie DR, Peterson BL, et al. Further analysis of trials with azacytidine in patients with myelodysplastic syndrome: studies 8421, 8921, and 9221 by the Cancer and Leukemia Group B. J Clin Oncol 2006; 24:3895–3903.

69. Fenaux P, Mufti GJ, Santini V, et al. Azacitidine (AZA) treatment significantly prolongs overall survival compared with conventional care regimens: results of the AZA-001 phase III study. Program and abstracts of the 49th Annual Meeting of the American Society of Hematology; December 8–11, 2007; Atlanta, GA. Abstract 817.

70. Lyons RM, Cosgriff T, Modi S, et al. Results of the initial treatment phase of a study of three alternative dosing schedules of azacitidine (Vidaza) in patients with myelodysplastic syndromes (MDS). Program and abstracts of the 49th Annual Meeting of the American Society of Hematology; December 8–11, 2007; Atlanta, GA. Abstract 819.

71. Dacogen™ (decitabine) for injection prescribing information, May 2006. Available at: www.dacogen.com/docs/pdf/dacogen-prescribing-information.pdf. Last accessed February 19, 2008.

72. Saba HI, Lübbert M, Wijermans PW. Response rates of phase 2 and phase 3 trials of decitabine (DAC) in patients with myelodysplastic syndromes (MDS). Blood 2006; 106:2515.

73. Van den Bosch J, Lübbert M, Verhoef G, Wijermans PW. The effects of 5-aza-2'-deoxycytindine (decitabine) on the platelet count in patients with intermediate and high-risk myelodysplastic syndromes. Leuk Res 2004; 28:785–790.

74. Lübbert M, Wijermans P, Kunzman R, et al. Cytogenetic responses in high-risk myelodysplastic syndrome following low-dose treatment with the DNA methylation inhibitor 5-aza-2'-deoxycytidine. Br J Haematol 2001; 114:349–347.

75. Kantarjian H, Oki Y, Garcia-Manero G, et al. Results of a randomized study of 3 schedules of low-dose decitabine in higher-risk myelodysplastic syndrome and chronic myelomonocytic leukemia. Blood 2007; 109:52–57.

76. Saunthararajah Y, Nakamura R, Wesley R, et al. A simple method to predict response to immunosuppressive therapy in patients with myelodysplastic syndrome. Blood 2003; 102:3025–3027.

77. Saunthararajah Y, Nakamura R, Nam J, et al. HLA-DR15(DR2) is overrepresented in myelodysplastic syndrome and aplastic anemia and predicts a response to immunosuppression in myelodysplastic syndrome. Blood 2002; 100:1570–1574.

78. Barrett J, Sloand E, Young N. Determining which patients with myelodysplastic syndrome will respond to immunosuppressive treatment. Haematologica 2006; 91:583-584.

79. Jonásova A, Neuwirtovà R, Cermàk J, et al. Cyclosporin A therapy in hypoplastic MDS patients and certain refractory anaemias without hypoplastic bone marrow. Br J Haematol 1998; 100:304–309.

80. Berer A, Ohler L, Simonitsch I, et al. Long-term improvement of hematopoiesis following cyclosporine treatment in a patients with myelodysplastic syndrome. Wien Klin Wochenschr 1999; 111:718–818.

81. Shimamoto T, Tohyama K, Okamoto T, et al. Cyclosporin A therapy for patients with myelodysplastic syndrome: multicenter pilot studies in Japan. Leuk Res 2003; 27:783–788.

82. Ogata M, Ohtsuka E, Imamura T, et al. Response to cyclosporine therapy in patients with myelodysplastic syndrome: a clinical study of 12 cases in and literature review. Int J Hematol 2004; 80:35–82.

83. Dixit A, Chatterjee T, Mishra P, et al. Cyclosporin A in myelodysplastic syndrome: a preliminary report. Ann Hematol 2005; 84:565–568.

84. Matsuda A, Germing U, Jinnai I, et al. Difference in clinical features between Japanese and German patients with refractory anemia in myelodysplastic syndromes. Blood 2005; 106:2633–2640.

85. Atgam® (lymphocyte immune globulin, antithymocyte globulin [equine] sterile solution) full prescribing information. Revised November 2005. Available at: www.pfizer.com/files/products/uspi_atgam.pdf. Last accessed February 22, 2008.

86. Teramura M, Kimura A, Iwase S, et al. Treatment of severe aplastic anemia with antithymocyte globulin and cyclosporin A with or without G-CSF in adults: a multicenter randomized study in Japan. Blood 2007; 110:1756–1761.

87. Lim ZY. Low IPSS score and bone marrow hypocellularity in MDS patients predict hematological responses to antithymocyte globulin. Leukemia 2007; 21:1436–1441.

88. Yazji S, Giles FJ, Tsimberidou AM, et al. Antithymocyte globulin (ATG)-based therapy in patients with myelodysplastic syndromes. Leukemia 2003; 17:2101–2106.

89. Killick SB, Mufti G, Cavenagh JD, et al. A pilot study of antithymocyte globulin (ATG) in the treatment of patients with 'low-risk' myelodysplastic. Br J Haematol 2003; 120:679–684.

90. Molldrem JJ, Leifer E, Bahceci E, et al. Antithymocyte globulin for treatment of the bone marrow failure associated with myelodysplastic syndromes. Ann Intern Med 2002; 137:156–163.

91. Sloand EM, Greenberg P, Wu C, et al. Immunosuppressive treatment is associated with durable responses and a survival advantage in younger patients int-1 myelodysplastic syndrome. Blood 2005; 106:2519.

92. Sokol L, List AF. Immunomodulatory therapy for myelodysplastic syndromes. Int J Hematol 2007; 86:301–305.

93. Bartlett J, Dredge K, Dalgleish A. The evolution of thalidomide and its IMiD derivatives as anticancer agents. Nat Rev Cancer 2004; 4:314-322.

94. Raza A, Meyer P, Dutt D, et al. Thalidomide produces transfusion independence in long-standing refractory anemias of patients with myelodysplastic syndromes. Blood 2001; 98:958–965.

95. Thomas D, Estey E, Giles F, et al. Single agent thalidomide in patients with relapsed or refractory acute myeloid leukemia. Br J Haematol 2003; 123:436–441.

96. Zorat F, Shetty V, Dutt D, et al. The clinical and biological effects of thalidomide in patients with myelodysplastic syndromes. Br J Haematol 2001; 115:881–894.

97. Moreno-Aspitia A, Colon-Otero G, Hoering A, et al. Thalidomide therapy in adult patients with myelodysplastic syndrome. A North Central Cancer Treatment Group phase II trial. Cancer 2006; 107:767.

98. List A, Kurtin S, Roe DJ, et al. Efficacy of lenalidomide in myelodysplastic syndromes. N Engl J Med 2005; 352:549–557.

99. Raza A, Reeves JE, Feldman EJ, et al. Long term clinical benefit of lenalidomide (Revlimid) treatment in patients with myelodysplastic syndrome without Del 5q cytogenetic abnormalities. Blood 2006; 108:250.

100. Revlimid® (lenalidomide) prescribing information, March 2007. Available at: www. revlimid.com/pdf/REVLIMID_PI.pdf. Accessed February 21, 2008.

101. Runde V, de Witte T, Arnold C, et al. Bone marrow transplantation from HLA-identical siblings as first-line treatment in patients with myelodysplastic syndromes: Early transplantation is associated with improved outcome. Bone Marrow Transplant 1998; 21:255–260.

102. Sierra J, Pérez W, Rozman C, et al. Bone marrow transplantation from HLA-identical siblings as treatment for myelodysplasia. Blood 2002; 100:1997–2004.

103. Castro-Malspina H, Harris RE, Gajewski J, et al. Unrelated donor marrow transplantation for myelodysplastic syndromes: outcome analysis in 510 transplants facilitated by the National Marrow Donor Program. Blood 2002; 99:1943–1951.

104. Sutton L, Chastang C, Ribaud P, et al. Factors influencing outcome in de-novo myelodysplastic syndromes treated by allogeneic bone marrow transplantation: A long-term study of 71 patients. Blood 1996; 88:358–365.